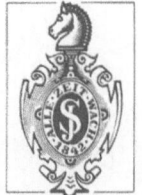

Société Internationale de Chirurgie Orthopédique et de Traumatologie

50 Years of Achievement
Paris October 10th, 1929 – Kyoto October 15th-20th, 1978

Edited by E. Vander Elst

Introduction by C. Casuccio

Springer-Verlag Berlin Heidelberg GmbH 1978

Edouard Vander Elst, M. D.
Avenue de Tervuren 194 A, Box 10
B-1150 Bruxelles

With 40 Figures

ISBN 978-3-662-38804-4   ISBN 978-3-662-39712-1 (eBook)
DOI 10.1007/978-3-662-39712-1

© by Springer-Verlag Berlin Heidelberg 1978.
Originally published by Springer-Verlag Berlin Heidelberg New York in 1978.
Softcover reprint of the hardcover 1st edition 1978

Typesetting and printing: Offsetdruckerei Julius Beltz KG, Hemsbach

2124/3140-543210

To
Floyd H. Jergesen
tenth President of S.I.C.O.T.,
who entrusted to me the task of preparing partly the celebration
of the fiftieth anniversary of the foundation of S.I.C.O.T., in the
hope that I do not and will not disappoint him.

VdE.

PROF. DR. PHILIPP ERLACHER
A 1130 WIEN XIII, GOBERGASSE 11—15
TEL. 82 11 97

Wien, 2o.3.1978

An den Herrn Präsidenten der S.I.C.O.T.
Prof. Casuccio
und den Herrn Präsidenten des Kongresses
Prof. Tamikazu Amako
An die Mitglieder des Büros des Intern.Komitees
der S.I.C.O.T.
und an die Teilnehmer des Kongresses !

Anläßlich des 5o jährigen Bestehens der S.I.C.O.T. erinnere
ich mich mit großer Rührung und Genugtuung an die Gründung
der S.I.C.O.T. in Paris 1929. Es bewegt mich um so mehr, als
ich mit Paul Lorthior als einzig überlebender Gründer von
den großen berühmten Namen übriggeblieben bin. Wir 21 Mitglieder waren damals in Paris gar nicht so überzeugt, daß
unser Versuch zu so einem weltweiten Erfolg führen würde,
aber ich bin jetzt sehr glücklich darüber.

Ich wünsche von ganzem Herzen noch viele erfolgreiche Jahre
für S.I.C.O.T. und einen vollen Erfolg dem Kongress in Kyoto.

DOCTEUR PAUL LORTHIOIR
PROFESSEUR HONORAIRE À L'UNIVERSITÉ

RUE EDITH CAVELL, 32
1180 BRUXELLES

TÉL. : 43.33.00

Bruxelles, le 24 mars 1978

Messieurs les Présidents,
Mesdames, Messieurs,
Mes Chers Amis,

S'il est un souvenir inoubliable dans ma carrière médicale, c'est celui de la soirée d'Octobre 1929, au cours de laquelle fut fondée, à l'hôtel Grillon à Paris, la Société Internationale d'Orthopédie (ce n'est que bien des années plus tard que la Traumatologie fut ajoutée à son patronyme).

Je me trouvais à cette réunion avec les représentants les plus prestigieux de l'Orthopédie.

Beaucoup d'entre eux furent mes Maîtres - Beaucoup furent mes amis - Philipp Erlacher est avec moi le dernier des survivants et je me joins à lui pour former du fond du coeur les voeux les plus sincères pour la prospérité et la pérennité de la S.I.C.O.T.

Aux membres de la S.I.C.O.T

Table of Contents

Introduction*

By C. CASUCCIO, *President of S.I.C.O.T.*

Presentation

The Société Internationale de Chirurgie Orthopédique et de Traumatologie (S.I.C.O.T.) is about to reach its first fiftieth year of life. In fact it was in the evening of October 10th, 1929, that twenty-one of the foremost orthopaedic surgeons in the world met in Paris and founded the "Société Internationale de Chirurgie Orthopédique" (S.I.C.O.)**.

In that very meeting the basic rules of the statutes were determined, in order to ensure the smooth running and the progress of the society; Sir ROBERT JONES, a name of great prestige, was appointed to the Presidency and VITTORIO PUTTI and HERMANN GOCHT were appointed Vice-Presidents; date and seat for the first congress were also fixed: June 5th and 6th, 1930 in Paris.

The first fiftieth anniversary of our society is an event well worthy of a special celebration. The International Committee which met in Copenhagen in July 1975 on the occasion of the 13th Congress, decided that the official celebrations should be held in the course of the 14th Congress, which will take place in Kyoto, Japan, on October 15th/20th 1978, and in that there should be an exhibition of documents, photographs and other material showing the salient facts of the fifty years history of the society.

Moreover, the International Committee decided that the jubilee should be marked by the publication of a commemorative volume. President JERGESEN (whose three years of presidency came to an end in Copenhagen) entrusted the treasurer of the society, EDOUARD VANDER ELST, with the task of editing the book.

---

* Manuscript received for publication August 3rd, 1978.

** The society was given the name "Société Internationale de Chirurgie Orthopédique" (S.I.C.O.). On the occasion of the 3rd Congress, held in Bologna in 1935, VITTORIO PUTTI who was chairing the congress, strongly upheld that it was time for a change of the name of the society by adding "et de Traumatologie". He had to overcome some opposition, but finally the whole assembly of the members approved the new name "Société Internationale de Chirurgie Orthopédique et de Traumatologie".

And now, as in Copenhagen I had the very great honour of being president of the society, and the honour is even greater since my presidency thus coincides with the celebrations for the jubilee, it is therefore my duty to present the work accomplished by our treasurer.

With modesty VANDER ELST states that "this historical outline is by no means complete and that there are a number of gaps that ought to be filled", and he also adds that "the main ingredient was my own enthusiasm for S.I.C.O.T.". Such words certainly capture the favour of the reader and lead him to a better appreciation of this historical review.

Reading the book one realizes how much effort the author put into editing the work. Even though he could collect a good quantity of information from the proceedings of the congresses and from the publications of the "Recueil Administratif" of more recent years, the information was certainly not sufficient. Therefore he must have searched in the archives of the society, asked for direct information, for papers, personal correspondence and so on, from those whom he presumed could give them to him. E. VANDER ELST has made an enormous effort to obtain documents of all sorts in the greatest number, in order to render his outline of the history of the society as complete as possible. In my opinion the author has fully succeeded and thus offers us a book full of information, precious for anyone interested in our society and the men who contributed to its progress.

I can assure E. VANDER ELST that his book is a real mine of information most of which is still unknown not only to the youngest members, but even to some of the oldest. I belong to the latter group and have participated in all congresses of S.I.C.O.T. (except for the one held in Amsterdam in 1948) starting from the third one in Bologna in 1936. The remembrance of this congress is probably the most vivid, since I attended as a very young assistant of my unforgettable master, VITTORIO PUTTI*.

In fact, my 42 years of participation in the life of S.I.C.O.T. are reason enough to entitle me to express here my very positive judgement on the work

---

* I don't think the value of E. VANDER ELST's work can at all be diminished if I remark here that, the report on the Bologna Congress, and the renaming of the society (which became Société Internationale de Chirurgie Orthopédique et de Traumatologie) ought to have been a little more complete. In fact PUTTI must be credited for the new name. E. VANDER ELST just mentions that "At the General Assembly of Bologna, the German members voted as a minority against the proposal to add "et de Traumatologie" to the title of the Society". The proposal had been brought in by PUTTI, as it clearly appears in the book of the proceedings of the "troisième Congrés de la Société Internationale de Chirurgie Orthopédique" – Bologne – Rome, 21–25 September 1936, on page 55 under "Réunion du Comité International" and on pages 64 and 66, under "Assemblée Générale Rapport du Secrétaire Général".

that E. VANDER ELST offers us and which I am sure will have great success with the members of our society. And in the hope that my words may interpret the feelings of all the members of S.I.C.O.T., I wish to express E. VANDER ELST my gratitude and the warmest congratulations.

Transactions that Lead to the Foundation of S.I.C.O.T. (1913–1929)

Although E. VANDER ELST's outline already contains more than one hint about the period that preceded the foundation of S.I.C.O.T., I am sure I shall not displease the author if I dwell on that subject in more detail.

Indeed I was fortunate enough to be able to use from V. PUTTI's archives – kept with some thousands of most precious old volumes which he collected in his extraordinary library at the Istituto Rizzoli in Bologna – a packet of documents concerning S.I.C.O.T. and which contained both correspondence and photographs.

The oldest of the letters of the packet is dated November 25th, 1913, that is sixteen years before the foundation! It is a letter written by ROBERT W. LOVETT from Boston, and addressed to HANS SPITZY in Wien and VITTORIO PUTTI in Bologna. The contents indicate that either some exchange of correspondence or a meeting of the three colleagues had already preceded the letter.

LOVETT reports on some inquiries he made about the international societies already existing at the time, and says he found an international society for surgery, one for genito-urinary surgery, another one for otology and finally one for dermatology. He presumes there were some others, but he had not proceeded further with his inquiries "thinking that this was quite enough to justify the need for an orthopaedic association". Moreover, having studied the statutes of those societies, he submits to his colleagues a suggested scheme of statutes for the International Society of Orthopaedic Surgery to be constituted.

LOVETT also writes: "...the Americans to whom I have spoken are very much interested and very enthusiastic, and will regard it as a decided honor to belong". He plans to delegate the president, the secretary and one member of the American Orthopaedic Association, as well as the president of the Orthopaedic Section of the American Medical Association and one representative from each of the two Western Orthopaedic Societies, to appoint candidates for membership. However he added: "but I should only submit to the International Committee those names I approved of. The National Committee's work would therefore be purely advisory".

3

After this LOVETT, in three long pages, concentrates on the question of having a review of the society, which in his view was indispensable, and which he tought he would like to call "The International Journal of Orthopaedic Surgery".

Along with some other considerations LOVETT also remarked: "It seems to me that we must offer men some return of their membership in the International Association, and although I believe that the standard should be so high that it would mean a great deal to any man to be a member, at the same time I think we must offer them some substantial advantages besides merely belonging".

He was also considerably worried about the financial side of printing a review. He says he "looked into the matter of getting support from some of the foundations, such as the Rockfeller Institute, but I find nothing very promising in the way of a subsidy. ... I have avoided doing anything about that. It seems to me that it would be necessary for us so far as possible to stand on our own feet".

From his letter we can see they had already set up an Executive Committee, the members being LOVETT, PUTTI and SPITZY, the latter acting as a secretary. Closing his long letter, LOVETT apologises for the delay in supplying the information he gives in his letter, due to his being "anxious to ascertain American sentiment".

I thought it would be interesting to quote all those details from LOVETT's letter since they are a document that, at such an early date, the progress of the dealings had already progressed so far that it appeared the launching of the new society was at hand.

The letter in question was followed by an exchange of correspondence between SPITZY and PUTTI. In spite of the fact that SPITZY thought LOVETT's suggestions were excellent, he delayed any solution pending the opinion of the Executive Committee of the German Society of Orthopaedics, which was going to meet in Berlin. In fact, in another letter dated July 8th, 1914 SPITZY informed PUTTI that the Executive Committee had authorized him to carry on the dealings with him and LOVETT, and moreover that LOVETT had written he was going to travel to Europe and wished to meet his two colleagues around the end of July or the beginning of August. PUTTI answered back at once (13th July 1914) eager for the meeting and suggesting a few suitable places in Italy. He himself would have liked Courmayeur, at the foot of Mount Bianco, or perhaps Misurina, "a wonderful spot near the border between Italy and Austria". These are his words: "I don't know whether LOVETT and you are mountaineers: I am fond of alpinism, and think that from those spots we could organize some wonderful excursions that might take our minds off the serious worries for the International Society of Orthopaedics". And he adds: "I shall go tho the meeting taking along besides the opinion of the best Italian orthopaedic surgeons, my good legs and all my equipment for alpinism".

In PUTTI's dossier this exchange of letters stops in July 1914, and therefore I cannot know whether the planned meeting ever took place. Another series of letters starts again in July 1929, and in order to fill that long gap it may be worth while quoting from a speech PUTTI personally addressed at the opening meeting of the Bologna Congress (22nd September 1936). After he had expressed his thankfulness for the honour bestowed on him by appointing him chairman of the congress, he said*: "I imagine this is the way you have chosen to show me your appreciation for the success of this society *which I have been the first and the most convinced promotor of.* In this regard let me point out something which may be of some relevance in the history of our society.

Going back to 1913, in the course of a conversation I had in London with two eminent colleagues, now both deceased, ROBERT LOVETT from Boston and ROBERT JONES from Liverpool, I suggested the timeliness, in order to contribute to a more rapid progress and a wider spreading of orthopaedic studies, of creating a society that would bring together all those devoted to orthopaedics throughout the world. The proposal was consented to with keen interest, and a scheme of statutes was already being prepared when the World War broke out and interrupted all our plans.

The idea was seriously taken up again in 1923, in the course of a second meeting I had in Boston with LOVETT and JONES, but even that time it had to be set aside because of LOVETT's unexpected death**.

"Convinced as I was of the rightness of the cause, I was but waiting for a new occasion to resume the design. The occasion did occur in London in 1929 when the American Society and the British Society of Orthopaedics met at a joint congress presided by ALBEE. I then expounded the whole idea to ALBEE, and it was a special merit of the rapid and strong action undertaken by this eminent colleague from New York if, within a few months, the foundations of the society were laid and the first congress could be summoned in Paris on 2nd October 1930."

---

* what follows is a translation of the quotation given in Italian in the Book of Proceedings on p. 10.

** ROBERT WILLIAM LOVETT, born in Beverly, Mass., on 18th Nov. 1859, died in Liverpool on 2nd July 1924 in the house of his old friend Sir ROBERT JONES. He taught orthopaedics at the University of Harvard, Boston.

In confirmation of PUTTI's words I found two letters addressed to him by FRED H. ALBEE, which are worth being quoted almost totally.

July 29th, 1929. "In accordance with our understanding I am sending the enclosed letter to the following men. I presume your letters have also gone out by this time and sincerely hope you will be in Paris on Oct. 10th." A list of 31 names follows. And here are the contents of the letter forwarded to the 31 colleagues a list of which he had given to PUTTI:

"Dear Doctor...

During the recent conjoint meeting of the British Orthopaedic Association and the American Orthopaedic Association, held recently in London, the question of the advisability of founding an International Orthopaedic Association came up spontaneously, and was discussed informally by a group including Sir ROBERT JONES of England, Professor PUTTI of Italy, Dr. MURK JANSEN of Holland, and Dr. GOLDTHWAITE and myself from the United States. It was unanimously agreed that such an association should be organized. The suitable time and place for an organization meeting were also considered. Professor PUTTI suggested Paris as the most central place, and October 10th as the earliest and most suitable date.

It is needless to emphasize the opportunity for cooperation and exchange of ideas between the various nations which such an organization would effort. The success of the meeting in London is a good augury for the succes of the projected association. I am sure you are in favour of it in a general way, and I hope that you can arrange to take an active share in its organization in Paris, at the Hotel Crillon, October 10th.

I am hoping for an early and favourable reply."

On receipt of ALBEE's circular of July 29th, with the invitation to the organizing meeting at the Crillon Hotel on Oct. 10th, HARRY PLATT – Sir HARRY today – wrote PUTTI a letter (Aug. 9th, 1929) informing him he had talked to Sir ROBERT JONES and to BRISTOW, whom ALBEE had also invited to take part in the scheduled meeting in Paris, and the three of them were convinced "that things are moving rather too rapidly". HARRY PLATT went on saying that the question had been discussed by the Executive Committee of the British Orthopaedic Association in the first months of that year and, though on the whole they approved of an international association, it was decided things should proceed "very slowly". Furthermore October 10th was not a convenient date for Sir ROBERT, for BRISTOW, and for himself either, and the same was for some other old members of B.O.A., who in any case ought to be present when the new association would be launched. The letter closed with a request in Sir ROBERT's name, who was away on holiday, "to try and hold things back if possible". Sir HARRY also wrote: "I spoke to him this morning, and he is quite definite in his view that it would be wiser to hold a preliminary meeting at a later date and at a more convenient time".

PUTTI answered PLATT that, as far as he was concerned, he was willing to give up the fixed date for a later one to meet in Paris, but the enterprise was to be considered as already launched, and it would have been very difficult to go back again. The only possible alternative was to meet in Paris and discuss the basic principles of the new society informally and not officially.

But a second letter from ALBEE to PUTTI, dated Sept. 3rd, 1929, came to remove any uncertainty. Here is the almost full text of it:

"Following your suggestion that we both write to certain men in different parts of the world in reference to the organization of an International Orthopaedic Association I have gone forward and done so. ... I have had almost 100% enthusiastic replies from everybody else, except Sir ROBERT JONES and his friends. Sir ROBERT is enthusiastic, but wishes to delay matters, while I am absolutely opposed to delaying the matter any longer. There are so many that can go to Paris on Oct. 10th that it seems an excellent time to get together and talk over the proposed organization. If we cannot completely consummate this organization at that time, it can be delayed till some later time. Sir ROBERT counsels us to discuss it in our various national associations. I am very much in favour of getting a representative group together in Paris.

If we can organize, I am very much in favour of your good self being the first president, and I would favour Sir ROBERT JONES being President Emeritus if you think it wise*. Please reply by cable if you can be present in Paris at the Hotel Crillon, October 10th."

Therefore, in spite of the attempts to delay matters, the meeting did take place at the date fixed by ALBEE and PUTTI, October 10th, at the Crillon Hotel: it started at 9 p.m. and was closed at 2 a.m. next morning. According to the minutes drawn on later indications by J. DELCHEF – who had been appointed Secretary General, but was absent being ill – after a resumé of the discussions PUTTI officially declared the International Society of Orthopaedics was established. The orthopaedic surgeons participating in the meeting were thus considered the founder members.

---

* As a matter of fact, Sir ROBERT JONES and not PUTTI was appointed president, evidently because of PUTTI's generosity in this situation.

In the night between October 10th and 11th, 1929, the history of the "Société Internationale de Chirurgie Orthopédique", that later became "et de Traumatologie", began.

I believe that PUTTI and ALBEE, two of the greatest orthopaedic surgeons we have had, well deserve having a place of honour in the list of the founder members. The former for his persevering endeavours, starting from 1913 up to the day the society was constituted, as well as for everything he did in favour of this creature of his for the rest of his life. He died when he had just reached his sixtieth, on Nov, 1st, 1940. The latter because, though he entered the scene but a few months before the foundation of the society, he must be credited for making the project his own the very moment PUTTI explained it to him, and consequently led it to a successful conclusion by his rapid and firm action. "I am absolutely opposed to delaying the matter any longer". This sentence of his shows his unyielding will to reach the goal as quickly as possible.

Even the names of SPITZY and LOVETT are worthy of being remembered above the others, although the latter died before he could enter the society which, with such warm enthusiasm, he had wished to see soon realized.

Notes on the Activities in the Triennium 1975–1978

E. VANDER ELST's work ends with the Copenhagen Congress, which was held in July 1975, that is 46 years after the foundation.

In my view the years between 1975 and 1978 also deserve to be mentioned in this history, at least to call attention to the fact that the activities of S.I.C.O.T. have not merely been restricted to the preparation and the proceedings of a congress every third year. Since it is in the wishes of the Executive Committee that this book should be presented at the 14th Kyoto Congress, it will obviously not contain a report of the congress itself. However, this history should cover the time up to July 1978, which is the time when the proofs will be passed for printing.

The colleague who one day (and perhaps it will be when the society has reached a century of life?) will take up again this outline in order to continue E. VANDER ELST's work, will have to start from the Kyoto Congress, which I suggest we call the Jubilee Congress.

After the Copenhagen Congress the most important fact worth being pointed out is the substitution of the proceedings of the congress with a new journal, named "International Orthopaedics".

It consists of four issues a year, the very first one of which appeared in January 1977. The journal is intended to contain the most important scientific contributions given at the congress together with other unpublished works by members and non-members of the society. Each work is carefully selected and is subject to the positive judgement of more members of the Editorial Board.

The purpose of having a journal which appears regularly is both to give our members and orthopaedic surgeons in general some scientific information at high level of interest, and to recall the liaisons between S.I.C.O.T. and its members more frequently than we used to in the past years, when the only contacts between congresses were just through the Books of Proceedings.

One serious objection to this effort can be made: the proceedings offered a thorough view of the importance of the congress and the way it developed, with not only the accounts of the scientific papers but also reports of the opening and the closing ceremonies, administrative sessions, and of all discussions, etc., while these details will be missing starting from the Copenhagen Congress.

Such a gap may probably be filled by printing a general report of the congress in the "Recueil Administratif". In any case the Executive Committees are convinced that publishing "International Orthopaedics" is indeed a most important innovation in the life of our society.

The main credit for this enterprise is undoubtedly to be given to R. MERLE D'AUBIGNÉ, who is now Honorary President of the journal. However, let me also ascribe part of the merit to the efficient members of the Bureau (ROBICHON and DHOLAKIA, Vice-Presidents, DE MARNEFFE, Secretary General, VANDER ELST, Treasurer, and WAGNER, Editorial Secretary) who succeeded in putting the idea into practice after facing and overcoming a number of serious difficulties connected with the publication of a journal, the first of which was the financial question. Last but not least we ought to remember with thankfulness those who undertook the heavy task of editing the journal: TAILLARD, Chairman, WAGNER, Editor, EVRARD and LOWE, Associated Editors, and all the members of the Editorial Board and of the Scientific Advisory Board.

With regard to "International Orthopaedics" E. VANDER ELST writes that as early as shortly after the first Paris Congress (Oct. 2nd–4th, 1930) the question of issuing a journal was raised. He remembers that on 25th Nov. 1930 ALBEE wrote to the president, Sir ROBERT JONES as follows: "We feel that a journal would be better than typewritten mimeographs reports, even it is only issued every six months". He thus concludes that if a group of persons must be credited for having given birth to an official journal of our society,

"International Orthopaedics", in January 1977, we must also give merit as well as honour to the group of orthopaedic surgeons who felt the need for an official paper already when the society had been just started.

I should like to stress E. VANDER ELST's statement reminding that, indeed, as early as in 1913, when he was having the very first contacts in view of constituting an International Association of Orthopaedic Surgery, LOVETT was already studying in every detail the possibility of issuing a journal, as he considered it indispensable (see p. 4). We must honor the memory even of this great colleague, who passed away before the society could be founded.

A very important change of the last three years which should draw the attention of those who are responsible for the future of S.I.C.O.T., is the phenomenon which has rapidly grown, of the birth of various international societies for superspecialized sections of our discipline. Evidently on one hand this fact is to be much appreciated as a sign of the vitality of our science that has developed up to the point of meeting the necessity of subdividing into sections, so that today we can have orthopaedic surgeons singly, or almost singly devoted to the surgery of the hand, foot, hip, knee, lumbar spine, paediatric orthopaedics, scoliosis, osteosynthesis, tuberculosis, arthroscopy, or merely to the scientific field of the specialty. On the other hand, however, the flourishing of superspecialized societies produces a number of problems which the Executives cannot fail to consider. The most important of all the various orthopaedic associations, S.I.C.O.T., is bound to defend the integrity of the science it represents and to avoid that the superspecialized societies should end by totally detaching from the discipline which created them.

In the course of the last three years the Bureau of S.I.C.O.T. has given close and thorough attention to the question of the relations between the mother discipline and what we might call satellite specialties.

Our Vice-President, ROBICHON, has been particularly devoted to this problem, the importance of which none should overlook. Contacts with the Executives of the superspecialized societies, who are practically all members of S.I.C.O.T. as well, have successfully established liaisons. Particularly it was agreed with some of the main ones that they should hold their congresses one or two days before, or after, S.I.C.O.T. Congress and in the same place. This will happen, for instance, with the "International Hip Society" which will have its first open scientific meeting in connection with the S.I.C.O.T. 1978 Congress in Kyoto the day before its starting date, that is on October 14th. Some other satellite societies have agreed to offer a particularly interesting session within the programmes of the S.I.C.O.T. Congress. For our next congress, this will be the case of sessions devoted to Paediatric Orthopaedic Surgery, Hand, Hip Surgery, Scoliosis, Traumatology, and research (organized by the new Société Internationale de Recherche Orthopédique et de Traumatologie (S.I.R.O.T.)). We all see that as a very important innovation in the organization of our congress, which will be further improved in the future.

Orthopaedics in developing countries is a problem to wich S.I.C.O.T. has arttached great importance in the last few years. A new society was recently founded named World Orthopaedic Concern (W.O.C.), an international society for Orthopaedic education and care in developing Countries. This new society manifested its intention of being linked with S.I.C.O.T. and is expecting some help from its Vice-President. DHOLAKIA during this triennium, has acted as an intermediary between the two associations and has contributed to a more efficient action in favour of orthopaedics. In developing countries this action will certainly be continued by the components on the new bureau who will be elected at the Kyoto congress.

The writer of these Introduction to E. VANDER ELST's work, with sincere regret called the attention of his Colleagues of the Bureau to the fact that in the course of fifty years of life efforts were never made to constitute a permanent foundation, or some awards and scholarships. Only the Organizing Commitee of the Tel Aviv Congress in 1972 offered 15 awards to scholars all over the world of either the clinic and the scientific fields of orthopaedics and traumatology. The award consisted of reimbursement of travelling and accommodation expenses. The organizers of the Kyoto Congress are now going to follow the example given by the Tel Aviv Congress: 6 awards, consisting of travelling expenses to Kyoto and return and free accommodation for the whole period of the congress, will be offered to scholars of orthopaedics and traumatology under 35 years of age.

In a letter I addressed at the end of December 1975 to all members of S.I.C.O.T. after some brief and basic information on the main problems on which the Executive Committee would have concentrated in the course of the triennium 1975–78, I expressed my hope and ambition that we might be able to give special relief to the celebrations of S.I.C.O.T. Jubilee with the creation of permanent funds to finance:

a) triennial awards for those orthopaedic surgeons who best contributed to the progress of orthopaedics and traumatology in the three years previous to the congress;

b) scholarships for specialising young doctors preferably from developing countries.

11

I pointed out that, since ordinary S.I.C.O.T. budgets cover current management expenses and printing costs of the journal, other sources ought to be sought such as donations from either private persons or from public bodies. So long S.I.C.O.T. has been living on membership dues only, but if its action is to grow positively we shall want to collect the financial means for it.

I called upon the members of S.I.C.O.T. to do their best in favour of the objects S.I.C.O.T. is aiming at, and to make an effort to interest and involve wealthy friends, patients, public institutions and producers of orthopaedic equipment.

My appeal has not remained unlistened to, in spite of the difficult times we are living in and of the difficult economic situations in most countries of the world.

Thanks to the generosity of the MAURICE E. MÜLLER Foundation in Bern, the AO-International, the GALEAZZI Foundation in Milan under the chairmanship of ZERBI, and the heirs of GALEAZZI, it has been possible to draw up an agreement between S.I.C.O.T. and these foundations that enables us to grant two awards and two scholarships every third year on the occasion of the congress. The prizes will be awarded for the first time in the course of the celebrations for S.I.C.O.T. Jubilee in Kyoto, as follows:

1st. The FRITZ STEINMAN/S.I.C.O.T. Golden Jubilee Prize, sponsored by the MAURICE E. MÜLLER Foundation. It will be awarded to the author of the best scientific work in clinical traumatology. The amount is 10,000 Swiss Francs.

2nd. The AO-International/S.I.C.O.T. Golden Jubilee Prize: sponsored by AO International. It will be awarded to the author of the best original research work in orthopaedics and traumatology. The amount is 10,000 Swiss Francs.

3rd, 4th. The RICCARDO GALEAZZI/S.I.C.O.T. Golden Jubilee Scholarship, sponsored by the GALEAZZI Foundation, Milan. It will be awarded to graduated medical doctors of any nationality who intend to devote to the study and research of orthopaedics and traumatology. Age limit: 30 years. The amount of each scholarship is italian lires 1,500,000, plus six months free entrance to the courses at either the GALEAZZI Orthopaedic Institute or another institute in Italy.

The gratitude of all S.I.C.O.T. members and myself is for the generous donors, in the hope that their example may be followed by others.

Also I should like to mention I have received generous donations from two firms.

It is our wish that these donations should constitute the beginning of a special fund to be spent in favour of the scientific progress of orthopaedics

12

and traumatology. We express all our thanks to these two firms, having confidence that a less generic and more personally directed action with firms and producers will give favourable results in the near future.

I believe that scholarships and awards, and the newly started fund are indeed another remarkable event in the life of S.I.C.O.T. and I do hope my successors will be able to widen the track and make their actions in that direction a real success. For instance, we might imagine what it would be if every member offered as little as twenty dollars each, "una tantum", for the special fund: that would already make up a sufficient sum for some substantial enterprise.

In my view the means for different awards or for special enterprises outside ordinary management, might also be collected from the various activities of the congress. In any case, I believe that S.I.C.O.T.'s income must be increased by all means if we want – and personally I wish it were so – S.I.C.O.T. not be restricted to things of ordinary administration only.

At this point, to avoid any possible misunderstanding, I should point out, that is certainly not contradicting our Secretary General, whose words at the General Assembly in Copenhagen on July 10th, 1975*, were: "It must be well emphasized that our Bureau Officers, and more specifically the Mini-Bureau of Brussels, with the actual means we have, can do not more. We have done our best". While I can testify that no doubt "the Mini-Bureau of Brussels" have done the best, on the other hand, just because with the actual means we can dispose of it is not possible to do more, we should try to improve S.I.C.O.T. sources of income.

When we consider its scientific activity throughout its first fifty years of life, I am quite convinced we can assert without fear of being belied, that a great deal of the enormous progress orthopaedics and traumatology have made in the last half a century has been the fruit of the studies and work of members of S.I.C.O.T., the results of which were made known to the world through S.I.C.O.T. Congresses. This is not the place and time for me to mention even only some of the main ones: it will be sufficient for anyone to read E. VANDER ELST's book to be fully convinced on the fact.

Therefore we can say S.I.C.O.T. has succeeded in attaining the goals which the founders set themselves, and as they are clearly and synthetically indicated in Art. 1 of the statutes: "Son but est de contribuer aux progrés de la science par l'étude de questions ressortissant au domaine de la Chirurgie

---

* Recueil Administratif du XIII Congrés International de Chirurgie Orthopédique et de Traumatologie, pg. 258.

Orthopédique et de la Traumatologie" ("Its aim is to contribute to the progress of science by studies relating to the orthopaedic surgery and traumatology").

The members of the Executive Committee, of the International Committee, of the Board of Directors (recently instituted), as well as the members of the various national sections, of the commissions of studies, all those who have given their active participation in the congresses, and finally even all those members who have contributed by supporting S.I.C.O.T. with their faith in the aims it pursues and with their financial help, all can feel proud of the progress of S.I.C.O.T. and should consider the celebrations of the fiftieth anniversary as their own festivity.

When we talk of scientific progress we ought to talk of change too. The society has undoubtedly changed a great deal since its first congress in Paris in 1930. The number of members has risen from the original 81 to about 2200, plus approximately 480 emeritus members. The number of the countries represented has risen from 15 to 71. And it should be pointed out that the number of members has increased so much in spite of the strict selection effected by the special commission through the examination of the titles of the candidates suggested by the national sections, which reflects the growth of orthopaedics and traumatology.

The organization of the congress has considerably changed too. Practically every new congress brings about some innovation in order to keep the level of interest of the congress up with the times. Just to give an idea, I shall merely mention that at the Paris Congress the problems foreseen by the Agenda were two: 1. The treatment of the congenital dislocation of the hip in patients over 15 years of age; with 4 speakers and 11 participants in the discussions. 2. The treatment of traumatism of the wrist; with two speakers and three participants in the discussions. The agenda of the Kyoto 1978 Congress includes lectures, revues, scientific reports, symposia, roundtable discussions, audio-visual scientific presentations, scientific communications on free subjects, symposia organized by superspecialized societies, the presentation of communications from the winners of the Fellowship Competition, etc. Up to the end of July 1978 the secretariat of the congress has already received over 2,000 entries.

I have already mentioned some other meaningful changes about the activities of the triennium 1975–78, i.e. the official journal of S.I.C.O.T. "International Orthopaedics" with S.I.C.O.T. Bulletin which substitute the Books of Proceedings, the question of the superspecialized societies and the question of orthopaedics in developing countries, awards and scholarships. Other problems S.I.C.O.T. is also considering through its special commis-

14

sions, such as nomenclature, classification of diseases, audio-visual media, surgical implants, education, and research.

There is one particular change which I should emphasize that makes S.I.C.O.T. different from what it was in its early years. The first seven congresses were all held in Europe: only in 1960 did we succeed in organizing one outside Europe, and this was in New York, after which the society really grew into a world association. In 1969 the congress took place in Mexico City, in 1972 in Tel Aviv, and at long last we are now going to have one in Japan in 1978.

Since the aim is that S.I.C.O.T. brings together the most valuable orthopaedic surgeons and traumatologists from all over the world, it is mandatory to follow the principle that the congress is to take place in whichever country where a group of orthopaedic surgeons are prepared to undertake the task, the responsibility and the economic effort of organizing it – naturally they are subject to the statutes and the final decision is up to the General Assembly of the members.

And it is basic that the same principle of rotation is adopted with the new appointments to the various offices. We must make every possible effort to avoid the impression that S.I.C.O.T. is a European association as opposed to a world one. Let us not forget that its two strong supporters, ALBEE from the United States of America, and PUTTI from Europe, had attained the goal of establishing a world society.

After this brief and certainly incomplete view of the growth of S.I.C.O.T. and the main changes that have occurred in its activities, together with a few remarks on possible changes projected into the future, I should like to conclude this introduction paraphrasing VITTORIO PUTTI's words in his speech opening the 3rd Bologna Congress (Sept. 22nd, 1936), as they seem to me very much up to date: the "Société Internationale de Chirurgie Orthopédique et de Traumatologie" has become the highest assizes for our discipline, the body that spurs and animates our work, and the most tangible and concrete affirmation of our will to perfect and strengthen a branch of surgery that has widened its field of action daily, for the benefit of mankind and the progress of science.

As orthopeadic surgeons we must feel the pride of being members of such an institution, and as to the younger ones of us the goal and ambition of their careers should be that of being admitted to it.

I. Foundation*

10 October 1929, 10 p.m.
Hotel Crillon, 10 Place de la Concorde, Paris

In the course of the last two hundred years or so the Place de la Concorde and the buildings that surround it have witnessed a fair number of events, some happy, others tragic.[1] But on the evening in question for a particular group of men there was occasion only for joy, enthusiasm and hope; indeed, for orthopaedic surgeons all over the world. The Event was taking place.

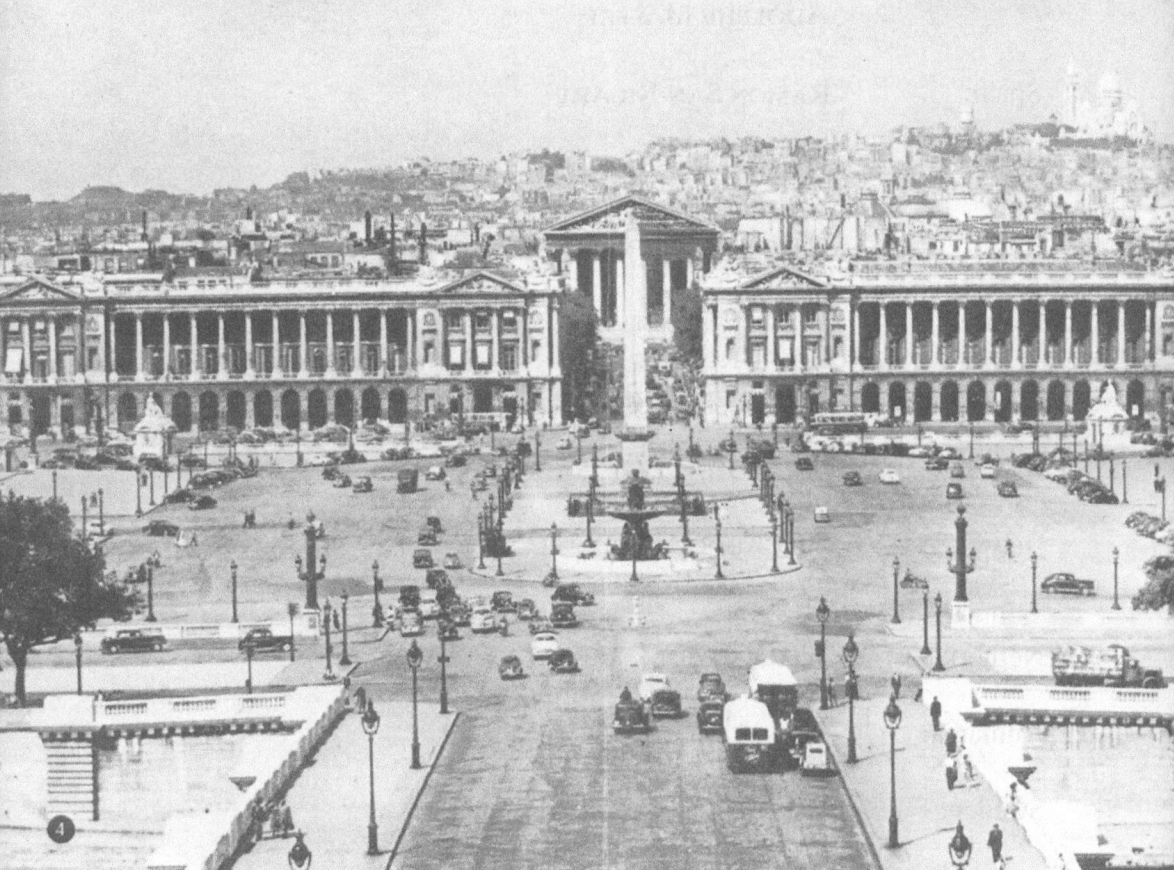

Fig. 1. This is the place! (B. YOUNG)

___
* Manuscript received for publication: April 1st, 1978.

Twenty-one men, inspired by courage and good will – and heaven knows, they needed it – were combining their resources to create the means to promote orthopaedic surgery and unite those who, the world over, devote their energies to this branch of surgery. Their objectives were progress and fraternisation.

At this juncture we should perhaps recall the names of these twenty-one courageous men, and the countries they represented[2]:

Austria:	PHILIP ERLACHER
	HANS SPITZY
Belgium:	JEAN DELCHEF
	PAUL LORTHIOIR
	ADOLPHE MAFFEI
Spain:	RAMON SAN RICART
United States:	FRED ALBEE
	WILLIAM BAER
	HENRY W. MEYERDING
France:	LOUIS OMBREDANNE
	LOUIS ROCHER
	ETIENNE SORREL
Britain:	Sir THOMAS A. T. FAIRBANK
Italy:	RICCARDO GALEAZZI
	VITTORIO PUTTI
Netherlands:	WILLEM MURK JANSEN
Rumania:	JEAN JIANO
Sweden:	PATRICK HAGLUND
	HENNING WALDENSTRÖM
Switzerland:	ALFRED MACHARD
Czechoslovakia:	JAN ZAHRADNICECK

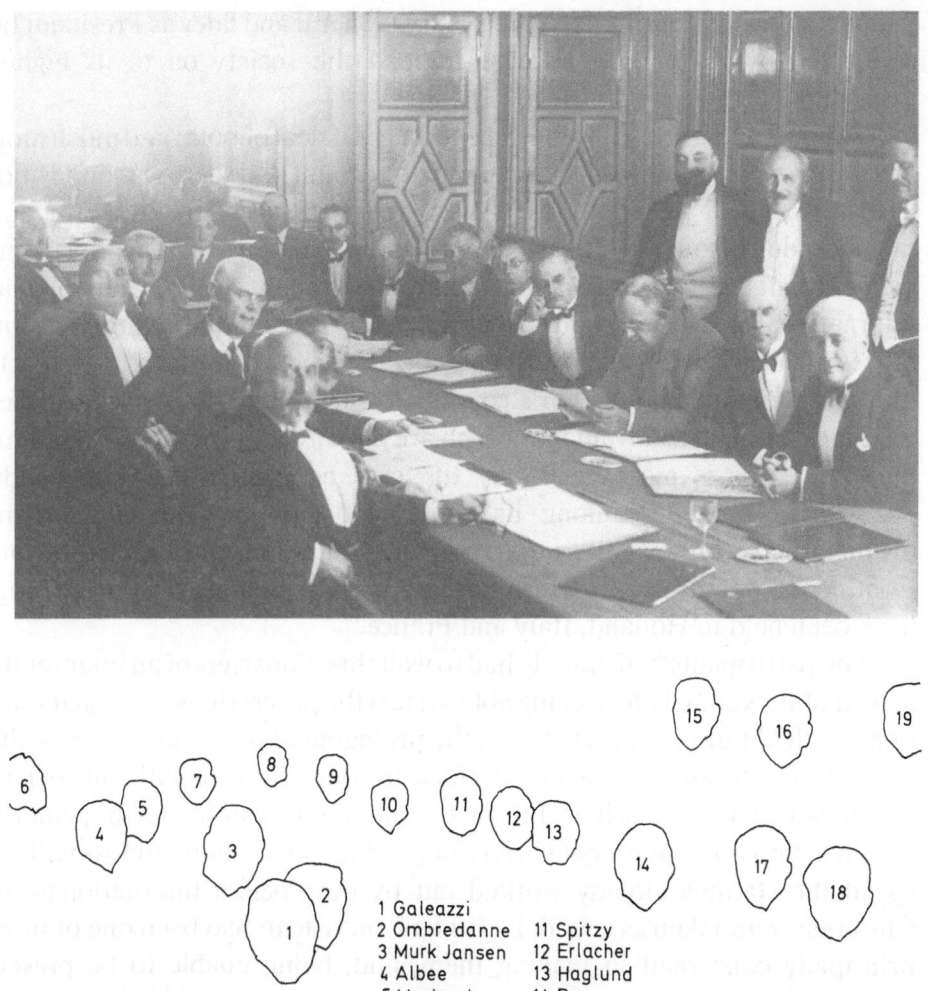

1 Galeazzi
2 Ombredanne
3 Murk Jansen
4 Albee
5 Machard
6 Zahradniceck
7 San Ricart
8 Meyerding
9 Lorthioir
10 Jiano
11 Spitzy
12 Erlacher
13 Haglund
14 Baer
15 Sorrel
16 Maffei
17 Fairbank
18 Putti
19 Waldenström

Fig. 2. The founders: the few to whom we owe so much

It is with great pleasure that we pay tribute to PHILIP ERLACHER and PAUL LORTHIOIR, who are still among us. Today they are the sole survivors of this esteemed group, those very few to whom is owed so much, to use a well-worn phrase. We would like to express in all humility our recognition of everything they have done. It should also be pointed out that in fact JEAN DELCHEF was not present on this memorable evening, since he was laid up with an attack of gout[1]. First as Secretary General and later as President he, supported by his colleagues, was to lead the society on to its highest achievements.

Courage and good will – they needed a great deal of both, and much more besides. For historical truth compels me to recount that there was opposition – from England – serious as it was well structured, in the form of a memorandum from the British Orthopaedic Association. This document explicitly stated two arguments militating strongly against founding an international society for orthopaedics: "... The multiplicity of existing Societies and Associations has already become a burden which threatens to become intolerable." (Author's comment: Already...) "... The projected association offers no advantages which are not alreadey provided by existing Societies. This is more especially the case as the British Orthopaedic Association numbers among its active and honorary members many distinguished orthopaedic surgeons, both in America and in various Continental countries..." During the last few years, successful meetings have been held in Holland, Italy and France.[3]

The participants had already had to wait three-quarters of an hour for the arrival of F. ALBEE before being able to start the proceedings[4,5] – and it was a bombshell. ALBEE and PUTTI were the protagonists in the discussion of this opposition*. In any case it was decided to found an international society, which was named Société Internationale de Chirurgie Orthopédique: S.I.C.O. Of course the new society needed a constitution, and so with all speed the statutes already worked out by the Société Internationale de Chirurgie were taken as a model. (JULES LORTHIOIR had been one of those principally concerned in making them, and, being unable to be present himself, had delegated his son, PAUL LORTHIOIR, to take his place.)

There are at least three reasons why it would be a grave mistake and a flagrant historical untruth to report this English opposition without further comment. The first is that Sir HARRY PLATT – whom we remember with great respect and warmth – in leaving his archives to us showed considerable fair play, which is just as much a British characteristic as the contrariety mentioned above. The second reason is also connected with Sir HARRY, in that for many years he had a great deal for the benefit and furtherance of S.I.C.O.T. Finnaly, without necessarily intending to, with their legendary sense of equilibrium the Britons doubtless helped to temper the ardour of some of their colleagues which might otherwise have got out of hand.

---

* The S.I.C.O.T. archives contain numerous letters to and from ALBEE which show beyond any doubt that he played a major part in founding the society. For reasons unknown he never held a leading position in it.

The meeting went on late into the night, reflecting the zeal of the participants and the heat of the debates; and even after the closure of the proceedings a few enthusiasts,[5, last §] put their first decisions down on paper, and these were to be the basis of the charter.

We should all pay tribute to these magnanimous and clear-sighted founders. Their magnanimity certainly went beyond all limits; to prove this I need only quote PUTTI's call for "... a small membership consisting of those present as charter members and gradually enlarging the organization, *the older men to lead the younger in serious work*";[5] or for "... *a more manageable and equally effective machine for progress and fraternisation*"* (letter from PLATT to ALBEE, Hotel Crillon, 8 October 1929, S.I.C.O.T archives). There are many more examples, as we shall see; but for the time being let us just recall that, after the difference of opinion mentioned above, the unanimous choice for president of the new association was Sir ROBERT JONES, undoubtedly the most eminent of all orthopaedic surgeons in the world at that time, but also a signatory to the aforementioned manifesto of the British Orthopaedic Association. Nor can we fail to be moved by the magnanimity and dedication expressed in the letter from Sir HARRY PLATT (same letter): "I should have liked immensely to come, if only to have a chat with you..." Let us once more pay tribute to Sir HARRY.

Our founders also possessed extraordinary vision. For too long orthopaedics had been confined to the "conservative" realm:[6] "cripples", patients with only one arm, with club foot or other handicaps, fell exclusively to the lot of bone-stetters, and then only with a certain degree of condescension. The repertoire of these latter, since the time of JEAN VENEL (1740–1791) had been limited to the use of corsets, shoes, various types of apparatus, chairs, and mechanical devices for remedials. Meanwhile tenotomy, osteotomy, amputation, osseous 'suture', remained exclusively in the domain of the surgeons – even before the advent of anaesthesia and asepsis/antisepsis. It was at the end of the last century that this yoke was finally cast off: between 1887 and 1926 national societies of Orthopaedic Surgery were established in nine countries: the United States, the Netherlands, Germany, Italy, England, France, Scandinavia, Belgium and Japan. Many others were to follow throughout the world. At last a whole multitude of problems which up to that time had been more or less consigned to oblivion were tackled and solved in a progressive and logical way. Congenital dislocation of the hip, more and more extensive osteotomy, fracture surgery, correction of discrepancy in the

---

* Author's italics.

21

length of limbs, arthrodesis, ankylosis and arthroplasty – and this list is by no means exhaustive – nothing seemed intractable or impossible any longer. It was especially in their recognition that the time was ripe to co-operate on a worldwide scale that the merit of these twenty-one founders lay; and much credit is due to them for this.

Their vision is no less evident in the statutes they laid down, which govern us to this day. Very little has been altered in the basic provisions agreed upon in the course of this auspicious evening[5], apart from a few additions and adjustments necessitated by the evolution of events and men.

Last but not least, many of these men grew to know and respect one another; virtually overnight they became firm and devoted friends*, which also became part of the tradition we inherited from them. It is indeed to S.I.C.O.T that many of us owe the opportunity of having come to know one another and become friends.

Progress and fraternisation were certainly noble and laudable objectives, but the creation of the means to achieving them had been laborious. There is no doubt that this difficult birth** had a good deal to do with the success that was to ensue. It is Law of Human Behaviour; and our twenty-one founders were human.

---

* The following day all were guests of Dr. YVONNE SORREL-DÉJERINE, in an atmosphere of cordiality and human kindness which was never to desert S.I.C.O.T.
** Letter from DELCHEF to PUTTI, 21 November 1929: "I have just returned from Paris where I encountered little enthusiasm for the new International Society of Orthopaedic Surgery..." (S.I.C.O.T. archives.)

II. Growing

A. First Congress:

Paris, 2–4 October 1930[7]

It took our valiant founders scarcely a year to get down to active business. Already they were organising the first congress, which was to bring together the international elite of the day in our field who, without running the risk of overstatement, may be considered part of medical and surgical history.[6]

The scientific work was begun in a brilliant inaugural session at the Amphithéâtre Vulpian[7], presided over by Sir ROBERT JONES, who held the offices of President of the Society and of the first congress. Having offered his thanks for the honour that had been done to him, he followed up most appositely by thanking FRED ALBEE: "The difficulties in gathering together the nations in friendly conference are prodigious. The task is surrounded by pitfalls. In this connection I would like to pay tribute to Professor ALBEE of New York for his vision, perseverance and tireless energy. We admire and congratulate him upon proving so important a factor in the birth of the International Society of Orthopaedic Surgerey." Sir ROBERT had entitled his address "The Domain of Orthopaedic Surgery".[8] It is a clear and concise analysis of the modern origins of our special field. It should be pointed out here that Sir ROBERT JONES had taken charge of the Manchester Ship Canal casualties before the First World War, and of the wounded of the British army during the war (with up to 30,000 beds). Moreover everyone knows of the part he and Agnes Hunt played in founding the Oswestry Hosipital for the handicapped. He was a man at the peak of his capabilities and in possession of a surpassing knowledge, the *primus inter pares*. Sir ROBERT's charm was legendary, and the following day at the Interallied Union banquet[8] "Sir ROBERT JONES (had) presided at the official Banquet, and in the single speech of the evening exercised his inimitable charm on all despite the linguistic difficulties".

Two subjects were on the agenda and the discussion was very animated. An account of this of some 180 pages appears in the first Volume of 'Proceedings'[7], which was to have twelve successors, and even at this early stage the question of publications arose. Hardly was the congress over when ALBEE wrote to Sir ROBERT JONES on 25 November 1930: "We feel that a journal would be better than typewritten mimeograph reports, even if it is

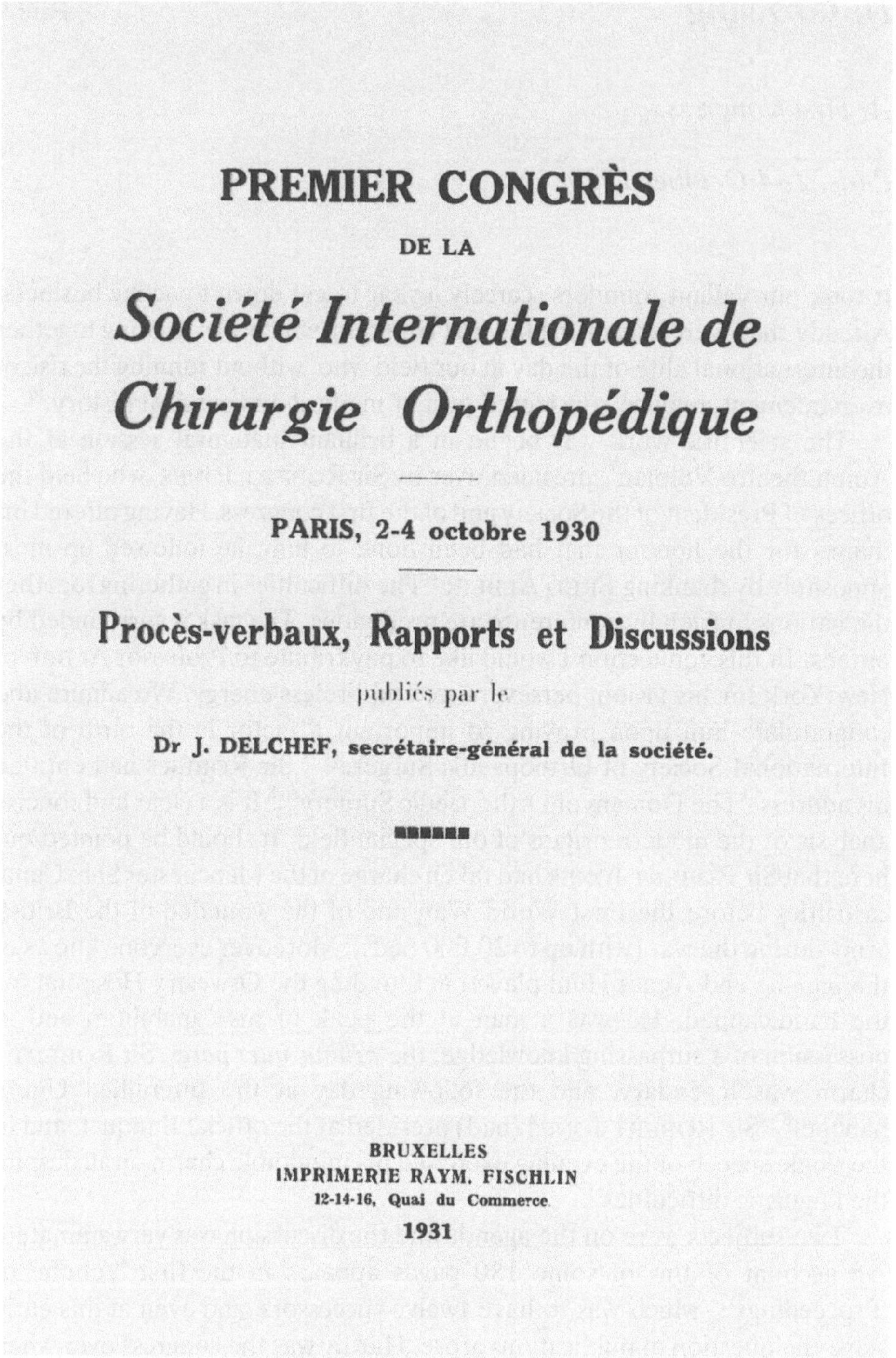

PREMIER CONGRÈS

DE LA

Société Internationale de Chirurgie Orthopédique

PARIS, 2-4 octobre 1930

Procès-verbaux, Rapports et Discussions

publiés par le

Dr J. DELCHEF, secrétaire-général de la société.

■■■■■■

BRUXELLES
IMPRIMERIE RAYM. FISCHLIN
12-14-16, Quai du Commerce
1931

Fig. 3. The very first proceedings of S. I. C. O. T. (at the time S. I. C. O.)

only issued every six months". With historical hindsight we can see that, whatever the merits and intuitions of those who were later to produce *International Orthopaedics* – i.e. the participants if the International Committee of Budapest in 1974* – the question had already been mooted in the earliest days of the society. In my view, therefore, it is only right to give due honour to both groups.

I have not been able to trace the number of participants in the first congress, or find a photograph of them. However, it is quite certain that there were already 81 members of the society and, even more significantly, three more countries had joined the nucleus of founder members: Cuba, Poland and Venezuela. Considering the difficulties of transport, or at least its relative slowness, this is a singular demonstration of the vitality of the organization and of the progress made in this short time. The leaders also had the insight not to wait any longer: *"La remise à un triennat de notre premier Congrès eut sans doute fait courir plus de risques à notre Compagnie ainsi exposée à l'oubli, l'indifférence".* (Postponing our first congress for three years would indubitably have entailed more risks, exposing our society to oblivion and indifference.)[7,p.19.] Last but not least, while steps had been taken to nominate the first reporters – and obtain their concurrence – the very day after the meeting at the Hotel Crillon, it was not until 21 February 1930, at the board meeting in London, that the decisions were made – and carried out – as this first congress shows.

There was further progress: Argentina, Hungary and Yugoslavia joined. Two other countries, Canada and Australia, also received agreement in principle. Thus the society became truly international, since 19 countries were, or were to be, represented in it. The future was viewed with confidence; the next congress was decided upon – the venue was to be London – and those who were to be responsible were delegated. *"Le prochain Congrès aura lieu à Londres en 1933. Il sera présidé par M. GABRIEL NOVÉ-JOSSERAND, de Lyon."* (The next conference will take place in London in 1933. It will be presided over by Mr. GABRIEL NOVÉ-JOSSERAND from Lyons.)[7,p.22]**

---

* At the instigation of ROBERT MERLE D'AUBIGNÉ, to whom, I must add, S.I.C.O.T. owes a great deal.
** It should be noted here that, S.I.C.O.T. has always had a President of the Society and a President of the Congress. With the exception of PUTTI, in 1936 in Bologna, the President of the Congress was always resident outside the venue of the Congress, which led to a certain lack of co-ordination. Since 1966 the President of the Congress has been a resident of the venue and has directed initial operations and organization (Statutes, Article IX, 2).

History continually repeats itself. In 1745 at Fontenoy, a little village in Belgium, the MARÉCHAL DE SAXE defeated the English in the presence of LOUIS XV. When the head of the English column halted at five paces from the French ranks, the officers saluted each other. "Order your men to fire", cried Lord HAY, the English captain. "No, monsieur, after you," replied the count D'AUTEROCHE. The incident was passed on to posterity in the charming but astringent phrase, "Après vous, Messieurs les Anglais!" The 'machine for fraternisation' was on its way, and the French and the English were trying to outdo each other in gallantry.

A final detail: "Operations were performed on two mornings by Professor OMBREDANNE and Dr. P. MATHIEU".[8]

First Congress: Paris, 2–4 October 1930

Officers

President:	Sir ROBERT JONES
Vice Presidents:	HERMANN GOCHT
	VITTORIO PUTTI
Secretary General:	JEAN DELCHEF
Treasurer:	ADOLPHE MAFFEI
Secretary of the Congress:	ALBERT MOUCHET

Reports

„*Behandlung der angeborenen Hüftgelenksverrenkung jenseits des 15. Lebensjahres*" (Treatment of congenital dislocation of the hip after the 15th year of age) by
LOTHAR KREUZ
F. J. GAENSLEN
Sir THOMAS FAIRBANK
VITTORIO PUTTI
"Traitement des traumatismes du poignet" (Treatment of injuries of the wrist) by
ALBERT MOUCHET
ALAIN MOUCHET
WILLEM MURK JANSEN

26

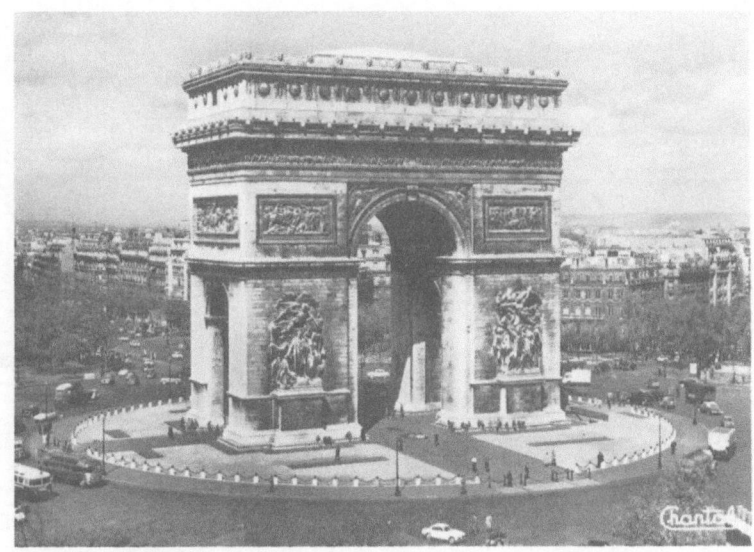

Fig. 4. It was (already) a triumph...

B. Second Congress[9]:   "Certitude"

London, 19–22 July 1933

The second congress of the new association should have got off to a joyous start; instead it began on a sad note, but not one of despair. The not altogether serried ranks, as constituted three years previously in Paris, were already losing strength; but reinforcements were on their way, just as vigorous and enthusiastic as the original cohort.

For three of the founders had died in the meantime: Sir ROBERT JONES, WILLIAM BAER and ALFRED MACHARD. At the same time we should mention JULES LORTHIOIR – and the members of the executive committee did not omit to do so – who had been a founder member by proxy, having sent his son PAUL LORTHIOIR to Paris.

At the time of the London congress S.I.C.O. already counted 216 members, 92 of whom were present. Reviewing the achievements of the

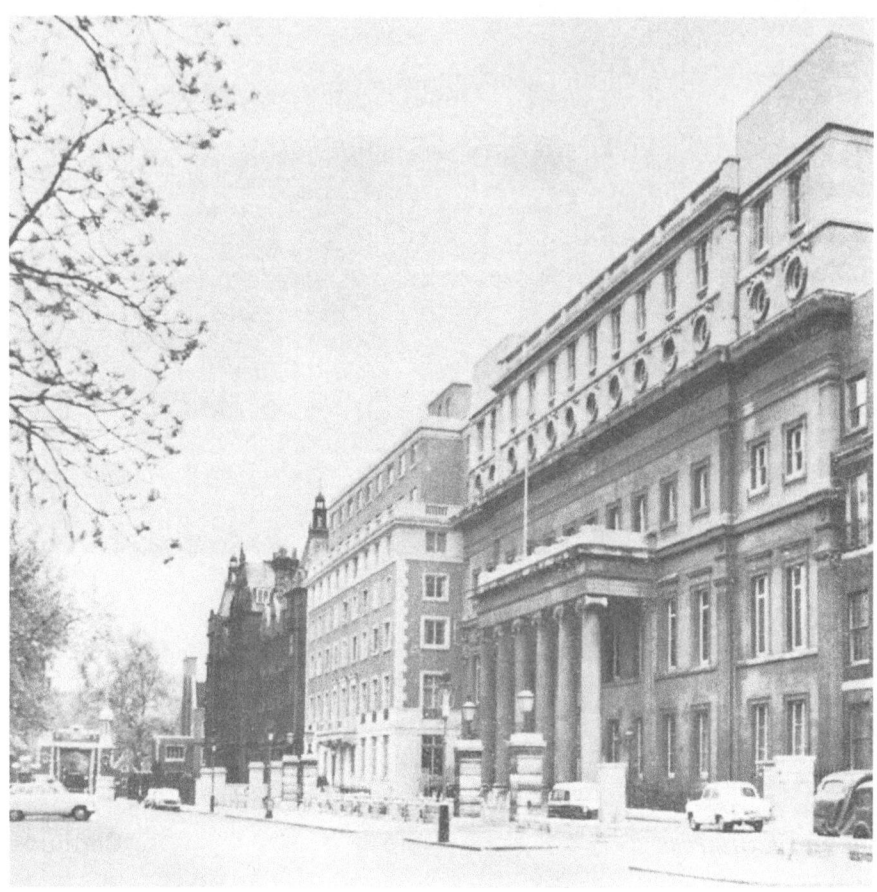

Fig. 5. The Royal College of Surgeons of England

society to date, the leaders were already able to show certain new developments: increase in the size of national contingents, expansion of congress programmes by the introduction of free papers on the two topics reported on. If we consider for a moment the variety of ways in which the programms of our modern congresses are presented (symposia, round tables, teaching conferences, brains trusts, etc.) we can only admire the vision of our predecessors. They had already conceived the new forms of congresses – and therefore of the furtherance of scientific knowledge – and went about implementing them without delay. The most appropriate way of giving some insight into their way of thinking is to reproduce the conclusion presented by the Secretary General to the International Committee:

28

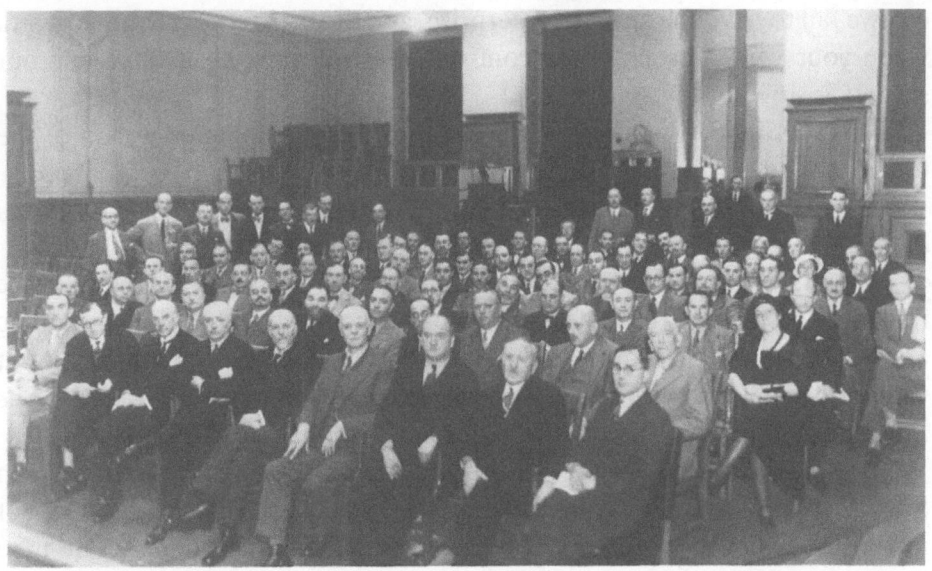

Fig. 6. The participants of the second meeting at the Royal College

Notre passé est garant de notre avenir. La route s'ouvre large, devant nous et nous n'avons pas le droit de nous arrêter. Nous nous devons de progresser et d'affirmer notre autorité, notre raison d'être dans le monde des Médecins qui ont les yeux tournés vers nous. Nous nous le devons, et nous le devons surtout à la Chirurgie Orthopédique, à cette Chirurgie de l'Appareil Moteur en train de s'individualiser dans la plupart des Pays, et dont notre plus beau titre de gloire est d'être les servants fidèles. Guillaume le Taciturne disait "Il n'est pas nécessaire d'espérer pour entreprendre, ni de réussir pour persévérer". Comment n'aurions pas, nous, l'esprit d'entreprise, la ferme volonté d'avancer quand, votre présence ici l'affirme, tous les espoirs nous sont permis, la réussite nous est assurée.

(Our past guarantees our future. The road ahead of us is wide, and we must continue along it. We owe it to ourselves to progress, and strengthen our leading position and raison d'être among the physicians who look to us. We owe it to ourselves, certainly, but above all to orthopaedic surgery, the surgery of the skeletal system, now in the process of becoming a field in its own right in the majority of countries, and which it is our great privilege to serve. William the Silent* said: "It is not necessary to hope in order to undertake a task, nor is it necessary to succeed in order to persevere". How

---

* Liberated the Netherlands (1533–1584) from the domination of the Spanish monarchy.

29

can we fail to have the spirit of enterprise, and the firm resolve to go forward, when your very presence here confirms that we are full of hope and our success is sure.)

This was indeed a superb profession of faith, a splendid vision of the future and an admirable programme.[9, p. 60]

The actual scientific work took up three full and fruitful days, and was divided into two parts of roughly equal importance.

The first part, presided over by GABRIEL NOVÉ-JOSSERAND, took place in the Barnes Hall of the Royal Society of Medicine. The President's opening address was a lucid account of the state of orthopaedic surgery throughout the world and it, too, was a profession of faith in the future: *"L'Orientation de l'Orthopédie en général"* (The orientation of orthopaedic surgery in general). We ourselves can see just how right he and JEAN DELCHEF were to believe in S.I.C.O.T., which had previously been known as S.I.C.O. There is plenty of numerical evidence of the advances made since the Paris congress: This time the 'Proceedings' ran to 616 pages in comparison with the previous 214. The two reports prompted 23 contributions to the discussion, while there were 23 free papers on the agenda. It is interesting to note that the first report was entitled *"Le Mécanisme des mouvements articulaires en général"* (The mechanism of joint movements in general). Surely an example of modesty – and a source of pride – to our modern biomechanicians. The second part comprised operating programms and visits to centres of orthopaedic surgery. Four hospitals were involved, and without in the least wishing to pass over the others, we should mention the Royal National Orthopaedic Hospital, which is well known throughout the world as one of the meccas of orthopaedic surgery.[10]

The social events proceeded in a like manner, surpassing those of Paris in 1930 – further evidence of the progress the society had made. The President of the congress and Madame NOVÉ-JOSSERAND invited the participants and their wives to a reception at a London hotel on 19 July. For all concerned it was a most pleasant opportunity for meeting their colleagues and friends from abroad in an atomsphere of cordiality. The following day, at the invitation of Sir HOLBURT WARING, President of the Royal College of Surgeons, the participants met in the famous building in Lincolns Inn Fields. Those many readers who know this edifice will have no difficulty in imagining the magnificence of the ceremony which, as you may have guessed, culminated in the conferring of the Honorary Fellowship of the Royal College of Surgeons upon the President of the Congress, GABRIEL NOVÉ-JOSSERAND. The visitors from abroad admired the treasures of the Royal College; the priceless collections, the splendid rooms, the magnifi-

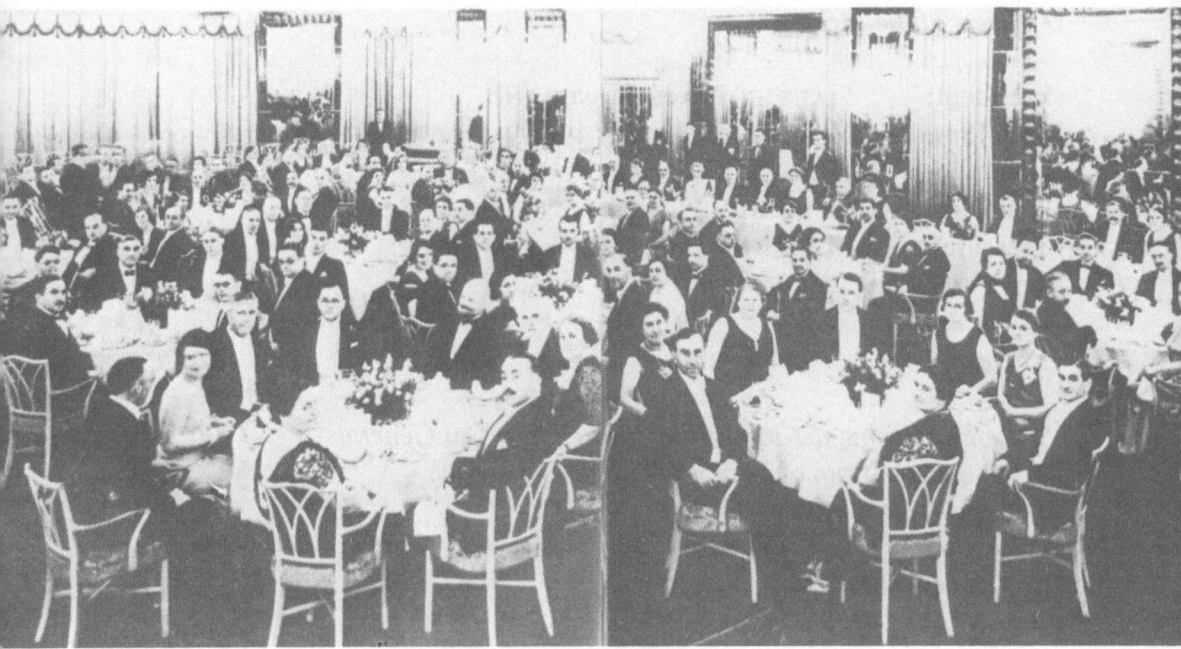

Fig. 7. The closing banquet at the Dorchester

cently andowed library and the picture gallery (containing paintings by the English Masters, e. g. HOGARTH, LAWRENCE, REYNOLDS and ROMNEY), which all had as their worthy guardian Sir A. KEITH, the Curator.[11]

Finally 150 guests gathered for the culmination of this second congress: a banquet held in a room of another London hotel. Sir WARREN LOW, President of the Royal Society of Medicine, opened the proceedings with typical British humour: "We live in an age of Congresses and Conferences. It is wonderful how our ancestors managed to do without them. There are, at this moment, in this City two Congresses on Medical subjects and only last week we finished another..." Sir WARREN continued in a more serious vein, at the same time paying tribute to all the great "orthopaedic" nations.

In his vote of thanks the President of the Congress, GABRIEL NOVÉ–JOSSERAND, did not omit to emphasize that the two greatest medical authorities in Great Britain at the time, Sir HOLBURT WARING, President of the Royal College of Surgeons of England[12], and Sir WARREN LOW, President of the Royal Society of Medicine of England, had honoured the meeting with their presence. At the close, the speaker announced the third congress, predicting "an even more resounding success" for it. This, as we shall see, was to prove to be true.

Officers of the Meeting

President: GABRIEL NOVÉ-JOSSERAND
Vice Presidents:VITTORIO PUTTI
                HERMANN GOCHT
Secretary: Sir HARRY PLATT
Treasurer: M. BROCKMAN

Reports

1. *Le Mécanisme des Mouvements articulaires en Géneral*
   (The mechanism of joint movement in general)
   HANS VON BAYER
   FRANCESCO DELITALA and SALVATORE CIACCIA
   RICHARD SCHERB

2. *Le Traitement des Coxites tuberculeuses*
   (Treatment of tuberculosis of the hip)
   PHILIP ERLACHER
   ADOLPHE MAFFEI
   MELVIN S. HENDERSON
   ETIENNE SORREL

3. Free Papers: 23

Officers of the Society
President: WILLEM MURK JANSEN
Secretary General: JEAN DELCHEF
Treasurer: ADOLPHE MAFFEI

Bologna and Rome, 21–25 September 1936[13]

The surprising thing we find in reconstructing the history of this congress is the sudden and exceptional improvement in all areas, right down to the smallest detail. It must be borne in mind that the society was only six years old, and those of us who are too young to have experienced these events must not forget that life did not afford the opportunities of all kinds which we take for granted today. Taking this into consideration, the quality of the work and the magnificence of the ceremonies appear all the greater.

The inaugural session was held in the ancient chapel of the Abbey of San Michele in Bosco, which houses the Rizzoli Institute: "The story of the foundation of the Instituto Rizzoli in Bologna has been often told – how an historic old Olivetan monastery on a hill in the ourtskirts of the city was purchased in 1880 by FRANCESCO RIZZOLI[14] and adapted for use as an orthopaedic hospital. RIZZOLI, who had at one time been professor of surgery in the university of Bologna, left his entire fortune for the conversion of the monastery to its new purpose and for its partial endowment."

Who could fail to be transported into an atmosphere of spiritual and scientific wealth in such a place? *Une foule compacte remplissait le vaste vaisseau. A la tribune et aux premiers rangs, chatoyaient les couleurs les unes vives, les autres sombres, des toges et des uniformes, relevés par l'éclat d'une pourpre cardinalice.*[13, p. 68] (A dense crowd filled the vast nave. In the gallery and in the front rows there was a wonderful play of the colours, bright and dark, of robes and uniforms, set off by a cardinals purple.)

There were a number of dignitaries present, representing all the authorities of the province. There were two short speeches, one by the mayor of the town of Bologna, S. E. TIENGO, and the other (in Latin) by Professor ALESSANDRO GHIGI, Rector of the University, on behalf of the authorities, followed by a speech of considerable energy by the President of the Congress, VITTORIO PUTTI. In his speech there is some very valuable information on the origins of S.I.C.O., and notably on the eminent role played from 1913 onwards by Sir ROBERT JONES and by R. LOVETT of Boston. As already metioned, it took the zeal and energy of FRED ALBEE to put the plans into practice. Subsequently PUTTI made a memorable plea on behalf of orthopaedic surgery and its recognition as a separate surgical entity.

33

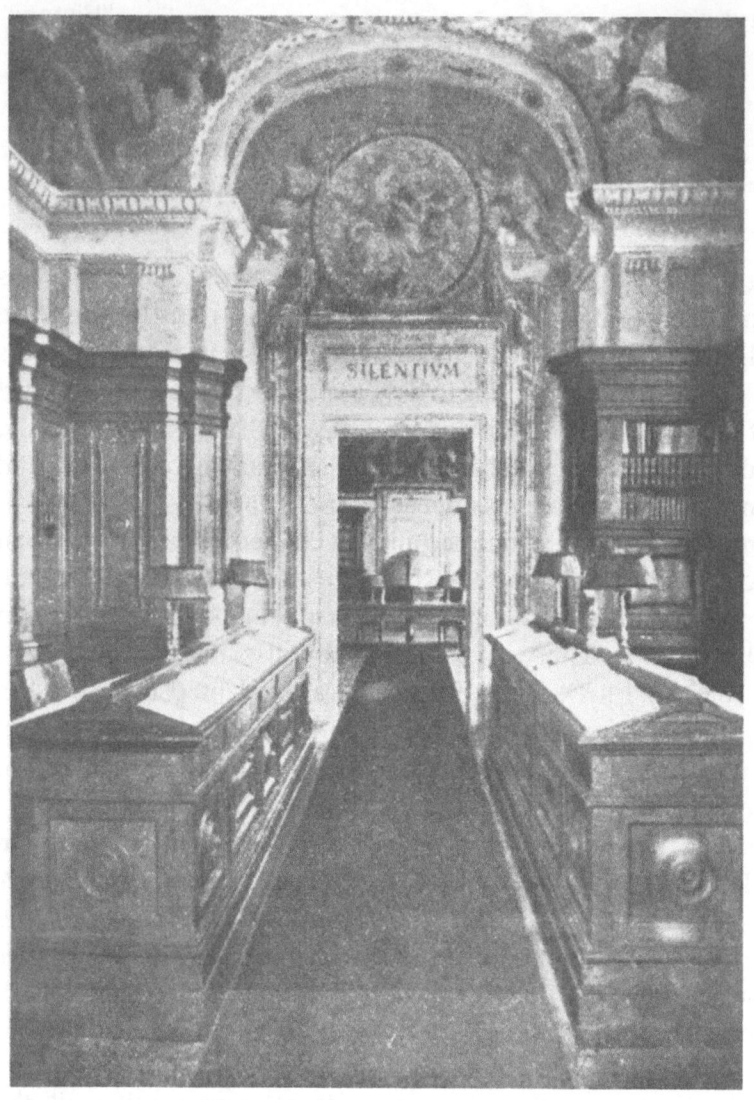

Fig. 8. The library of the Istituto Rizzoli, Bologna, formerly an olivetan monastery (with kind permission of J.B.J.S.)

And so to the work in hand. Two important questions were on the agenda; there were 20 contributions to the discussion on the first, and 24 on the second. This was followed by 30 free papers. The result of all this work: a volume of 726 pages.

34

It is in the activities of the International Committee that we find further proof of the dynamic energy which carried the society towards its goals, and of the confidence which motivated its members. At this time the society had 329 members from 28 countries; 121 members took part in this congress, and some of the had crossed the Atlantic, not only from the United States but also from Cuba and Argentina. Unfortunately 13 members had died since October 1929. *"Une des caractéristiques des organismes vigoureux est la réparation rapide de leurs pertes, la faculté de cicatriser aisément. S'inspirant de la Nature, les organisations humaines vivaces lui ont emprunté ses méthodes de conservation."* (One of the characteristics of healthy organisms is that they quickly make good their losses; their scars heal easily. Inspired by Nature, healthy human organisations have emulated her methods of conservation.)[13, Delchef, p. 39]

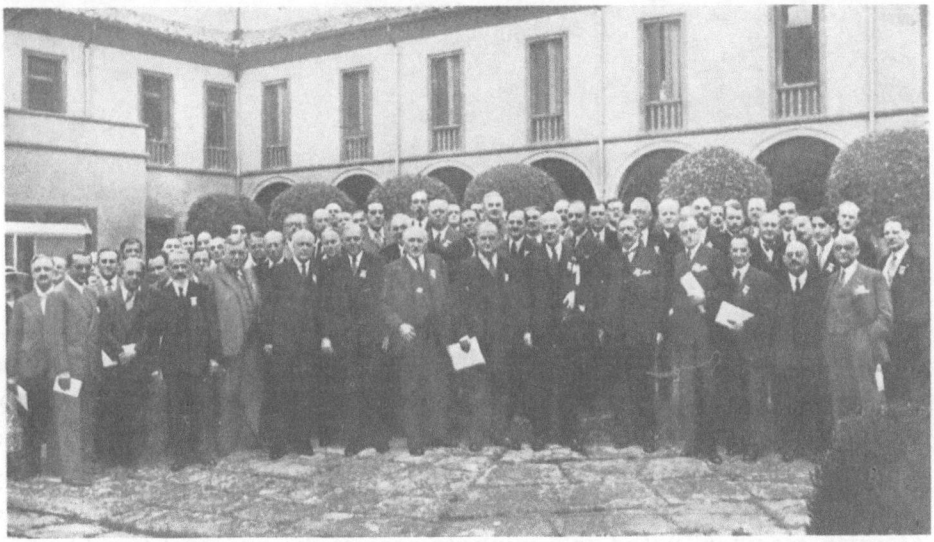

Fig. 9. The participants of the Bologna meeting in the courtyard of the Istituto Rizzoli

It was also in the course of this congress that the title and designation of our society was modified, with the word "Traumatologie" being added. This was an important detail; for in some countries traumatology remained in he hands of surgeons who refused obstinately to let go of it – and there is no evidence to suggest that this tendency has completely disappeared. In other countries the orthopaedists, having become surgeons in the way we have

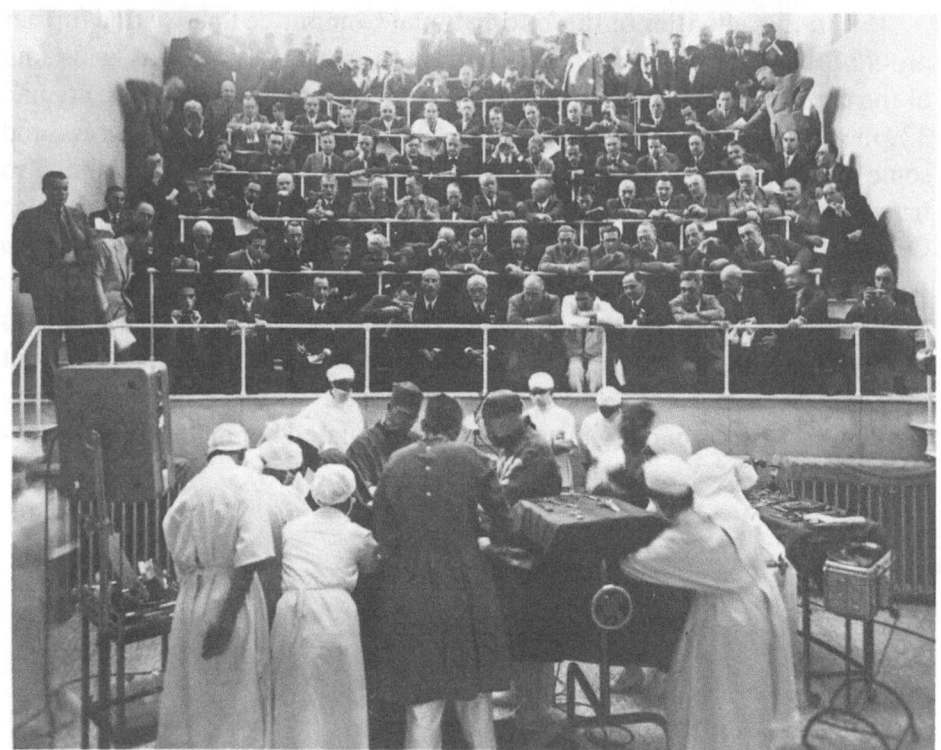

Fig. 10. PUTTI in his surgical Theatre

seen, only achieved recognition by limiting their practices to what may be termed "cold" surgery. They feared that by laying claim to the field of traumatology they might well once more become subservient to the surgeons. This was why the German-speaking orthopaedic surgeons, among others, opposed this change. "At the general Assembly at Bologna, the German members voted as a minority against the proposal to add *'et de Traumatologie'* to the title of the Society."[13] Nonetheless the motion was passed. Further demonstration of the growth of the society and the continued confidence in it: 75 new mebers were admitted.

Work carried on in Rome throughout the day of 25 October, and here, as at Bologna, there were operating sessions (under PUTTI in Bologna and under MARINO ZUCO in Rome). What appears to have been an innovation was a vast scientific exhibition, which was assiduously attended by the participants following the inauguration by PUTTI.

It is hardly necessary to add that the festivities and receptions were of the same quality as the scientific work, and in a way that only Italy, steeped in history, could offer: They were lavish. In Bologna on the evening of 21 September the President of the Congress, PUTTI, gave a gala dinner in the Great Hall of the Palace of the Podesta, resplendent with frescoes by the great artist ADOLFO DE CAROLIS. The President of S.I.C.O.T., L. OMBREDANNE, on behalf of the participants thanked PUTTI and those who had assisted him for their unforgettable hospitality, and Sir THOMAS FAIRBANK followed suit, speaking for his compatriots. PUTTI replied and in his turn thanked the civic authorities for their co-operation. Still on the subject of 'refreshment', the Podesta of Bologna held a reception for the participants the following evening, and the day after this the ancient Chapel of San Michele in Bosco was the scene of further revelries. PUTTI caused quite a sensation by having films made – and developed in record time – of a few characteristic moments of the meeting. By all accounts the chief attraction of the festivities was the visit of the wards and other buildings of the Rizzoli Institute.

PUTTI was a great collector of old books, a scholar devoted to cultures of the past, and nothing concerned with medicine, surgery and their past left him indifferent. He has been compared to HARVEY CUSHING[14], another famous collector and bibliophile. Incunabula, rare manuscripts, old instruments, famous paintings, frescoes discovered thanks to the scholarship of PUTTI himself; all this constitutes a treasury which, from all points of view, transformed the Rizzoli Institute into a mecca of orthopaedic surgery for the whole world.

History affords this particular benefit: it detaches a fact from its ephemeral contingencies and, being an exact science, "decants" the facts and deeds in order to give an account of the significance of the event. And so it was that B. MUSSOLINI gave audience to the participants of the congress at the Palazzo Venezia on 25 September at 2.30 p.m. The delegation consisted of about 50 participants, representing eight countries. Nothing more should be seen in this than a tribute paid to the leader of the government by his countrymen and their guests – a gesture of courtesy by persons of good breeding. The following account, perceptive and at times caustic, was penned by Sir HARRY PLATT. I know that may Italian colleagues and friends are far too discriminating to take offence at this; indeed I am sure that many of them would be disappointed to discover that I had kept this episode quiet, while they may now consider it 'released from the censor'. Here is Sir HARRY's text (Editorial, "Days remembered", in *Modern Medicine,* August 1971; i.e. Modern Medicine of Great Britain, Ltd):

Rome. September, 1936

It was a lovely September afternoon in Rome in the year 1936, and a number of members of the International Society of Orthopaedic Surgery (S.I.C.O.T.) had been warned to be ready to leave the afternoon scientific session before its completion. At a signal from a younger Italian colleague, we crept silently out of the amphitheatre to find a bus waiting for us. Already in the bus were a number of Congress Ladies whose passports, for some unknown reason, had been scrutinised two days before. All aboard, and the bus made its way through crowed traffic to the Palazzo Venezia. By this time, the secret was out. We were to be received by MUSSOLINI. We entered by a side door where a good looking high ranking officer in the Fascist Police glanced briefly at each one of us and bowed galantly to the ladies. Once in the Palace, we traversed salon after salon, all empty except for a young uniformed footman at each door. The late Sir THOMAS FAIRBANK, who used an old-fashioned hearing aid which involved carrying a largish black box, was halted by one of the young flunkies, obviously a country boy, who after some words of explanation allowed Sir THOMAS to continue his journey. We finally reached a large salon, again empty, where we were lined up under the leadership of our famous colleague Professor VITTORIO PUTTI of Bologna, whose sole concession to fascist costume was a black tie. Then through a door in the far corner there entered the Italian dictator, BENITO MUSSOLINI. He was greeted by a number of our Italian colleagues with the fascist salute and a cry of *"Il Duce"*. I regret to say that instinctively our right arms shot out with alacrity a few seconds later.* Il Duce shook hands with VITTORIO PUTTI, who, by the way, had treated one of his children for poliomyelitis. A few individuals were presented by name – our President, Professor LOUIS OMBREDANNE of Paris (whom I succeeded after the War) and our Secretary-General, JACQUES** DELCHEF of Brussels. Both have now passed on. Then Mussolini stuck out his chin – he badly needed a shave at 5.30 p.m.; his white duck suit was crumpled. He proceeded to welcome us, speaking in French with one false quantity only, as my friend Mrs. PHILIP WILSON of New York, herself Paris born, noted at the time. I remember that he asked us to look around and to note that Italy was prosperous and that everybody was working hard. He complimented us on the contribution we were making to the relief of disablement, and described us, not inaptly, as the

---

* According to other witnesses, the salute was not unanimous; probably Sir HARRY could asserve only those immediately next to him, since he was an eminent person in S.I.C.O.T. and therefore in the front row. (Note by VdE.)

** Obviously a misunderstanding; the correct first names were JEAN JOSEPH. (Note by VdE.)

engineers of the human body. He bowed, was saluted once more, then turned round and disappeared through the door by which he had entered. During the audience he showed no signs of nervousness. The year before, during the International Surgical Congress, he had been shot at by an English woman, who drilled a neat track through his nose. It occurred to some of us afterwards that he could easily have been eliminated during our audience in the Palazzo Venezia. But of course there would have been no escape for the assassin.

The final act of the congress now took place: a reception in the grounds of the Capitol, another centre of culture and art treasures, of natural beauty and harmony. Thus *"sur la colline d'ou l'Histoire ruisselle"* (on the hill whence History flows down)[13] this third and most memorable meeting of S.I.C.O.T. drew to a close. Who would have thought that ten long years of inaction were to be forced upon this admirable society, in its very prime? But for the time being we are only concerned to recapture the magnificence and surpassing productiveness of the third congress of S.I.C.O.T.

Third Congress: Bologna-Rome, 21–25 September 1936

Officers of the Meeting
President: VITTORIO PUTTI
Vice President: Sir THOMAS FAIRBANK
Secretary: OSCAR SCAGLIETTI

Reports

1. *"Les dérangements internes du genou"*
   (Internal derangements of the knee)
   KARL BRAGARD
   JOSÉ VALLS
   PAUL MATHIEU
   Sir HARRY PLATT
   LEON KALINA

2. *"Les arthrorises dans les séquelles de paralysie infantile"*
   (Arthrorises in the sequelae of cerebral palsy)
   LOUIS ROCHER
   CHRISTIAN ROCHER
   PIERO PALAGI

3. *Free Papers:* 30

Officers of the Society

President: LOUIS OMBREDANNE
Vice Presidents: HERMANN GOCHT
                    FRED ALBEE
Secretary General: JEAN DELCHEF
Treasurer: ADOLPHE MAFFEI

Appendix

Everything had been planned for a fourth congress in Berlin from 4–8 September 1939; World War II prevented it from being held. Let us nevertheless pay tribute to those who were selected to give reports and made the effort to prepare them. The S.I.C.O.T. archives contain offprints for:

1. *"Les résultats éloignés des réductions sanglantes et non sanglantes des luxations congénitales de la hanche"*
   (Long-term results of surgical and conservative treatment of congenital dislocation of the hip)
   BRUCE GILL: Treatment of congenital dislocation of the hip
   FRITZ SCHEDE: *Die Ergebnisse der unblutigen und blutigen Behandlung der angeborenen Hüftverrenkung*
   (Results of conservative and surgical treatment of congenital dislocation of the hip)
   OSCAR SCAGLIETTI: *Risultati della riduzione incruenta e cruenta della lussazione congenita dell'anca*
   (Results of conservative and surgical treatment of congenital dislocation of the hip)

2. *Le traitement des fractures du col du femur* (Treatment of fractures of the femoral neck)
   JOSÉ VALLS and ENRIQUE LAGOMARSINO: *El tratamiento de las fracturas del cuello del femur* (Treatment of fractures of the femoral neck)

40

N.B. LOTHAR KREUS, LOUIS TAVERNIER, ADAM GRUCA and SVEN JOHANSON were the authors nominated for other reports on the same subject.

Officers of the Meeting
President: GEORG HOHMANN (replacing HERMANN GOCHT, deceased)
Secretary: HELMUT ECKHARDT

Officers of the Society

President: LOUIS OMBREDANNE
Vice President: FRED ALBEE
Secretary General: JEAN DELCHEF
Treasurer: ADOLPHE MAFFEI

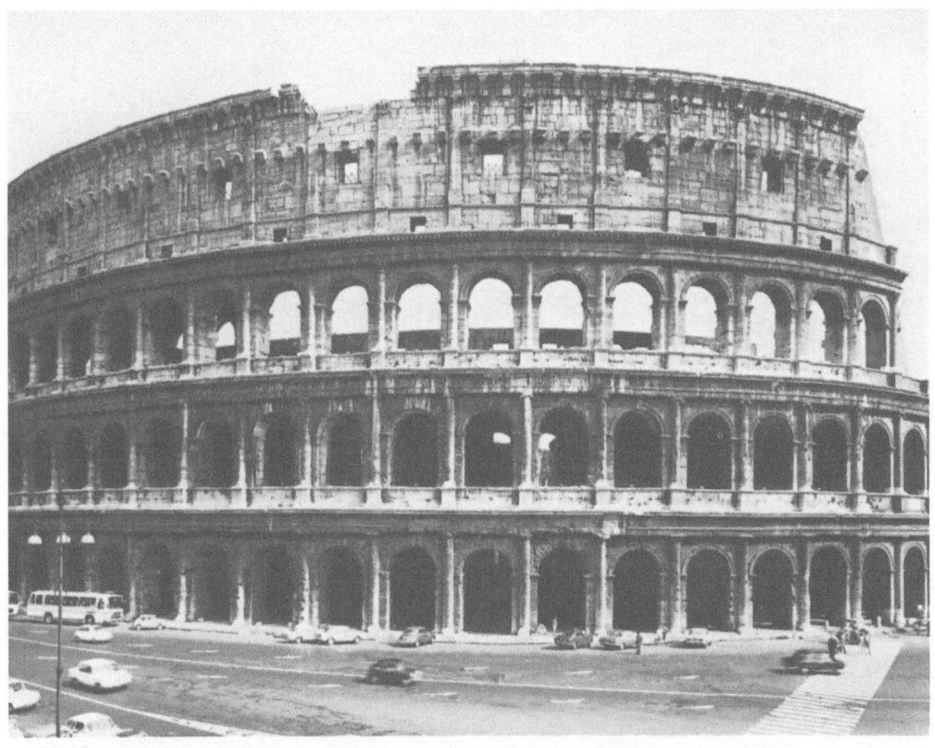

Fig. 11. The Coloseum in Roma, a symbol of S. I. C. O. T. 's energy

III. Revival: 1946

A. A Meeting in Brussels

The international association was scarcely ten years old when some dark clouds of a political and military nature gathered in the skies of Europe. S.I.C.O.T. was to be swept with the storm and forced into hibernation and inaction until it could be reborn seven years later. The society having been founded in Paris, it seemed appropriate to adopt the motto of that city: *"Fluctuat nec mergitur"*. Once more I can do no better than hand over the narrative to Sir HARRY PLATT; his keen humour and incisive pen are irreplaceable, and I would not wish to alter one iota: "At the Bologna meeting ... preliminary arrangements were made for the fourth Congress to be held in Berlin in September 1939 under the presidency of Professor HERMANN GOCHT with Dr. FRED H. ALBEE and Professor PATRICK HAGLUND of Stockholm as Vice Presidents. By July 1939 the programme was in the hands of all members, and most *"rapports"* on the main subjects had been printed and distributed. Many members had made travel arrangements. Professor GEORG HOHMAN of Frankfurt was in London in July with many of his Colleagues*, attending an international conference on "cripples", and he assured the late Mr. ROWLEY BRISTOW and this writer that no international incident would prevent the Congress being held. We had no reason to doubt this belief. But the meeting was cancelled."[15]

The war passed, and as is to be expected our founders had lost non of their enthusiasm or their confidence. JEAN DELCHEF, with his valiant soul and will of iron, renewed contact across the frontiers and in January 1946 eight men gathered in Brussels with as much energy and spirit of enterprise as they had shown in Paris in 1929. Some rather unpleasant files had to be opened due to the war, but the will to make a new start was so strong that the "machine for progress and fraternisation" set off again toward new goals which, as we know, were to be achieved with great success.

---

* On 1 September 1939 HERMANN GOCHT was the guest of JEAN DELCHEF at Coq-sur-Mer, at the Helio-Marin Institute (communication of JEAN DELCHEF, Jr. to the author).

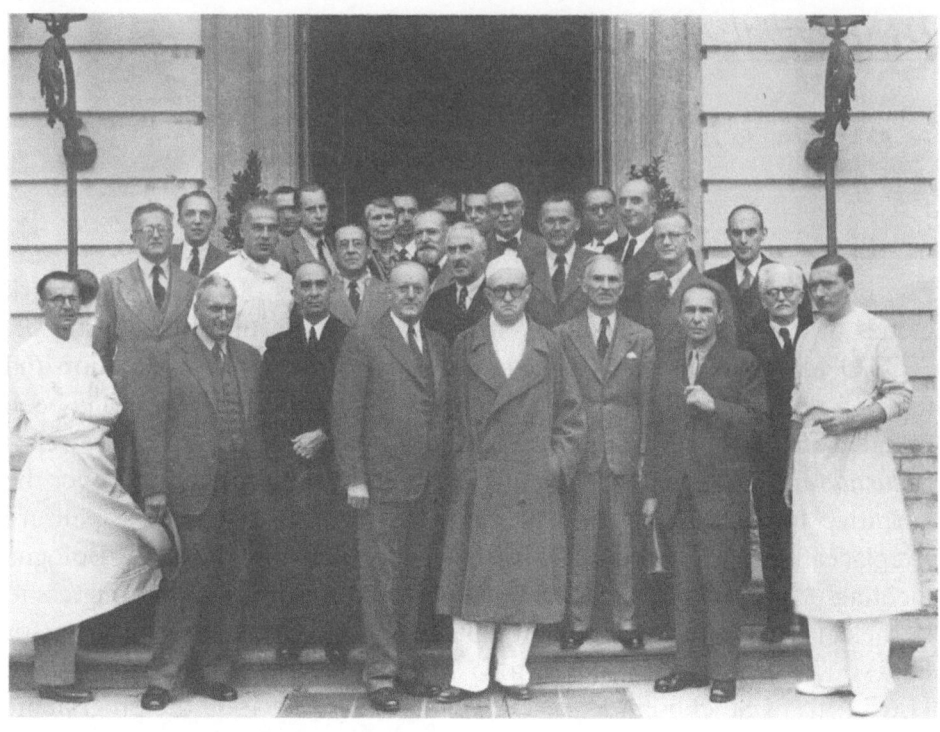

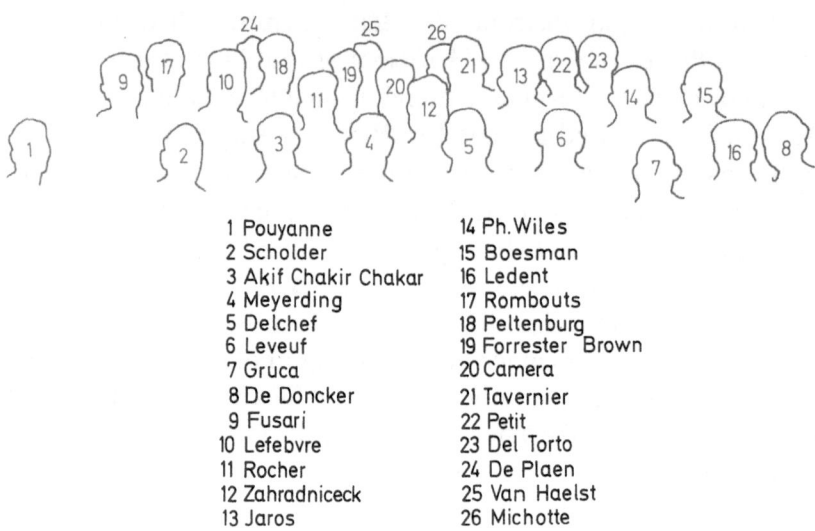

1 Pouyanne	14 Ph. Wiles
2 Scholder	15 Boesman
3 Akif Chakir Chakar	16 Ledent
4 Meyerding	17 Rombouts
5 Delchef	18 Peltenburg
6 Leveuf	19 Forrester Brown
7 Gruca	20 Camera
8 De Doncker	21 Tavernier
9 Fusari	22 Petit
10 Lefebvre	23 Del Torto
11 Rocher	24 De Plaen
12 Zahradniceck	25 Van Haelst
13 Jaros	26 Michotte

Fig. 12. When faithful friends meet again ... 5 october 1946 at DELCHEF's clinic

Sir HARRY, incontestably the unwitting historian of S.I.C.O.T., once again provides a faithful narrative. This is how in his inimitable humorous way he described the first stages of the revival.[16] This all took place in January 1946: "It was impossible for one whose last visit to the Continent was in the spring of 1939 to conceal his excitement as the Belgian coast and Flanders came into view through the windows of the Sabena* Company's twenty-seater plane. I turned to my neighbour, a young Belgian civil servant returning from an economic conference in London, and said: "This is D-day for me." "It will be rather different on this occasion," was his reply: "there will be no resistance."**

The Brussels airport looked dreary and empty in the darkening afternoon of a hard winter day. I was surprised to find the R.A.F. still in titular control and that all travellers went through the bottle-neck of British military security. At the Sabena office the wife*** of my Brussels friend and colleague – my hostess on many previous visits – was waiting with a car to convey me to the club of the Fondation Universitaire (F. U.) where I had been a temporary member on similar missions before the war. Behind its simple facade in the quiet Rue d'Egmont the interior of the F. U. looked as dignified and elegant as ever. Le tarif, allowing for the increased cost of living, was still moderate – English club prices for my room (the bathroom stocked with towels of pre-war quality) and for my "breakfast" (café complet). The table d'hôtel luncheon was a little expensive on British standards, but remembering the excellence of the pre-war cuisine this did not seem unreasonable. I was not disappointed.

The shadow international committee of eight**** people assembled next day, representing France, Great Britain, Scandinavia, Holland, and Belgium, and including the President of our International Association, one of the most distinguished of pre-war surgeons, now retired from his chair and hospital.***** Our business was to discuss plans for reviving the activities of the association, to decide when and where the next international congress should be held, and, most important of all, to expel members from enemy countries. After a three hours' sitting we had settled the rest of our business but failed to decide on the exact procedure of expulsion. The speed of arguments at times

---

*	Belgian Airlines.
**	Underground war.
***	Madame JEAN DELCHEF.
****	LORTHIOIR, BENTZON, SAN RICART, SORREL, HARRY PLATT, VAN ASSEN, OMBREDANNE and DELCHEF.
*****	LOUIS OMBREDANNE. (Notes by VdE)

left me giddy and guessing. At one stage, the torrential flow of French was interrupted by the Danish delegate* breaking into German, to be followed immediately by the Dutch and Belgians in the same language. As I had learned German at the age of nine, this was a welcome relief – but it was an ironical moment. The discussion was resumed later in the hospitable home of our senior Belgian colleague**, and before the large dinner party assembled in our honour had broken up. The Spanish delegate*** had arrived from Barcelona too late for our committee meeting but in time for the superb dinner. The proposition regarding expulsion was explained to him by our President in a sentence of incomparable brevity, possible only in the French language: "Nous cherchons une formule juridique valable."**** Shortly before midnight we had found the formula under "Article Onze" of the constitution, and we returned to the company and the cognac.

Next morning, a Sunday, I woke to find Brussels covered by a mantle of snow which rapidly froze on the pavements. The central heating of the F.U. was comforting, and I was loth to turn out in the evening to seek my dinner in a near-by restaurant. It was then that I came into contact with the prices of the universal black-market in food. For the first time in my life I argued with a waiter about the cost of a meal; we finally agreed on 150 francs (17s 6d) for the smallest lobster of a bunch arranged on a side table. The café filtre there, as in all the restaurants and cafés, was nectar. Next day the weather was savage and the sky dark. After settling my modest account at the F.U. I arrived at the Sabena office to be told that no plane could land at Croydon that day, though if the weather improved a special plane expected back from the Belgian Congo would leave early next morning. It was thus necessary to get accommodation for another night in Brussels in a hotel, where I met the full blast of the prices for tourists. I left the hotel at 6.30. next morning in pitch darkness in a "taxi noir" and was driven a quater of a mile to the now familiar Sabena office. "Soixante quinze francs monsieur – c'est le tarif du gouvernement." I protested that we had liberated his country at great cost, but paid up. The twenty-seater Congo plane left the icebound airport after a hazardous start. Our first attempt at a take-off was a failure – a mild bump –

---

*   BENTZON.
**   JEAN DELCHEF.
***   SAN RICART.
****   An attempt at translation: "We are looking for an adequate formula from the legal point of view."
(Notes by VdE)

46

back to earth just as we were airborne. We crossed the Channel at 3000 feet, in a beautiful sea of white clouds, to touch down at Croydon just three minutes before a dense fog enveloped the whole aerodrome."

In actual fact the eight leaders of S.I.C.O.T. showed great wisdom in postponing the decision on the expulsion of certain members. In any case they had made their point, showing that they were fully aware of the gravity of the question, and pre-empting accusations of indifference or negligence. Politics and Science should always be independant of each other, even if a few black sheep slip into either domain. We can only admire the moderation of these eight delegates, who succeeded in maintaining a most difficult balance.

A further decision was made[17,p.5], taking up the torch which had remained unextinguished since 1936: "... *respecter la cadence trienniale des réunions et fixer en conséquence le prochain Congrés en 1948. Toutefois, il parut inopportun de remettre à cette date les premières assises de la Société plongée en léthargie par les évènements. Une réunion dite de 'reprise de contact' fut décidée et fixée à Bruxelles les 2 et 3 octobre 1946"* (... to respect the triennial nature of the meetings and therefore to arrange the next congress for 1948. Nevertheless it seemed inappropriate to leave the next meeting of the society until that date, forced into inaction as it had been. So a meeting for 'Renewal of Contact' was decided upon, and fixed for 2 and 3 October 1946 in Brussels.)

And so it was.

B. Renewal of Contact: "Renaissance"

Brussels, 2–5 October 1946[17]

Owing to the events still fresh in everyone's mind, administrative matters rather outweighed questions of science. The International Committee, on which 15 countries including Italy and Austria were represented, made on decision in principle which was a masterpiece of moderation and tact: Concerning the legal files connected with the war, they decided that each member was to be judged according to his attitude and his deeds. The application of the measures was to be deferred until the signing of the peace treaty with Germany. The suggestion came from the French, formulated by the President, L. OMBREDANNE.* Again, we can only admire the tact of the President and the courtesy of the Assembly.

Then the stream of life reasserted itself, and three further countries were admitted: Iceland, Mexico and Turkey. *"Semper ad astra"* certainly seems to have been everyone's motto. The venue for the 1948 congress was chosen: Amsterdam. Two questions were put on the agenda, and the reporters were nominated. New candidates were approved, bringing the total membership to 382. A new classification was introduced, the Emeritus, which was conferred upon 28 members. Alas, by a cruel but natural balancing mechanism the long list of demises[17,pp.9–89] had claimed a further 45 members in the meantime. We should especially remember those of our founders whose names appear on this tragic list: FRED H. ALBEE, VITTORIO PUTTI, PATRICK HAGLUND, and above all ADOLPHE MAFFEI, who died heroically in Belsen on 20 February 1945 after a personal calvary which lasted three years.

On the scientific level, only one question was retained: functional improvement in amputees; and it was the privilege of G. PERKINS of London to introduce the debate, which was very lively, since there were no less than 19 contributions to the discussion. The meeting concluded with the presentation of 21 free papers. Seventy members were present as well as a large number of Belgian guests. An operating session was carried out by JEAN DELCHEF at the Neerijsse Clinic, which many of us subsequently came to know. Another was presented at the St. Pierre Hospital by the indomitable R. SOEUR, while a demonstration of prostheses was organised by G. HENDRIX, who has died, and by P. KEMPENEERS, who is still among us.

The social events were discreet but of a high quality. The President and Madame OMBREDANNE gave a reception on 12 October in the rooms of the Taverne Royale, a vibrant centre of Brussels life which is no longer there

---

* A final word on this rather awkward and delicate question: The Stockholm Congress (1951) decided to reinstate the German members. The decision was by no means unanimous, but once more the "machine for progress and fraternisation" was able to proceed on its way… It is only fair, and indeed vital to historical truth, to add that certain German members paid dearly for their scientific independance; for example, HANS VON BAEYER, expelled from the Heidelberg University Clinic at the time when he represented the spearhead of research into orthopaedic surgery (personal communication to the author from MATHIAS HACKENBROCH).

today. The participants gathered for a banquet by subscription on 3 October in the Town Hall. On 4 October, Dr. VANDE MEULENBROECK, mayor of Brussels and a most charming and pleasent man, did the honours at the Town Hall in his capacity as both colleague and host. The splendours of the Town Hall are well known to anyone who has spent a few hours in Brussels. There were interludes of music and drama. As for the ladies, the had been able to visit a place pervaded by the spirit of genius: the House of Erasmus; and also the museums of Brussels.

Like a traveller who has rested to regain his strength after a long and dangerous voyage, S.I.C.O.T. set out once more on its victorious journey. Of course new difficulties and problems would arise, but S.I.C.O.T. would always find capable and judicious leaders to guide it.

Officers of the Society

President: LOUIS OMBREDANNE
Secretary General: JEAN DELCHEF
Treasurer: CHARLES PARISEL
Second Secretary: ANTOINE BAILLEUX

IV. Flowering

A. Fourth Congress:[18]

Amsterdam, 13–18 September 1948

"The fourth congress of S.I.C.O.T. was held in the famous Indisch Instituut, Amsterdam, during the week September 13 to 18, 1948, under the patronage of her Majesty Queen WILHELMINA. Two hundred delegates attended from twenty-seven countries. The congress owed much to the Dutch capacity for smooth organisation, which was personified by the secretary, Dr. J. D. MULDER. On several occasions the president of the Congress, Dr. HENRY W. MEYERDING, expressed his relief that more trouble had not arisen in the timing of the sessions which on paper were filled, and indeed hopelessly overfilled, with vast numbers of contributions.* One of three days of scientific procceedings was devoted to reports on closed fractures of the spine, another to arthritis deformans of the hip joint, and a third to a series of short papers.

---

* R. MERLE D'AUBIGNÉ told me the following anecdotes:

"This great post-war congress had aroused considerable interest due to the long interruption (12 years, since the 1939 congress had been cancelled) and above all in view of the opportunity for the Europeans to meet their Ango-Saxon colleagues. One of the subjects was the treatment of osteoarthritis of the hip joint. Smith Petersen whose cup sent the audience into dream, had only agreed to speak on conditions that he was allowed 90 minutes. The committee agreed; the reputation of 'Pete' and the prestige of victorious America met with no resistance.

However, certain other speakers, who had not been warned, reacted in rather spectacular ways. PAUL MATHIEU, of Paris, spoke after Smith Petersen, and was allowed only 15 minutes. When the green light lit up after 14 minutes his voice quavered. But when the president gave the red light, Mathieu's face turned a similiar hue ... and remained so after the light went out. A few seconds later he stopped abruptly and scribbled a few words on a scrap of paper, which he handed to the president: his resignation from S.I.C.O.T. .... and he left the room.

PAUL MAGNUSSEN, of Washington, was on the programme for the same session, shortly afterwards. He was allotted 10 minutes, and was to be followed by less known speakers. With supreme calmness he outlined his main ideas and then added, "Well, gentlemen, anyone who wishes to hear about my experiences and results may follow me into the adjoining room, which I have reserved for one hour." And he left the room – followed by three-quarters of the auditorium.

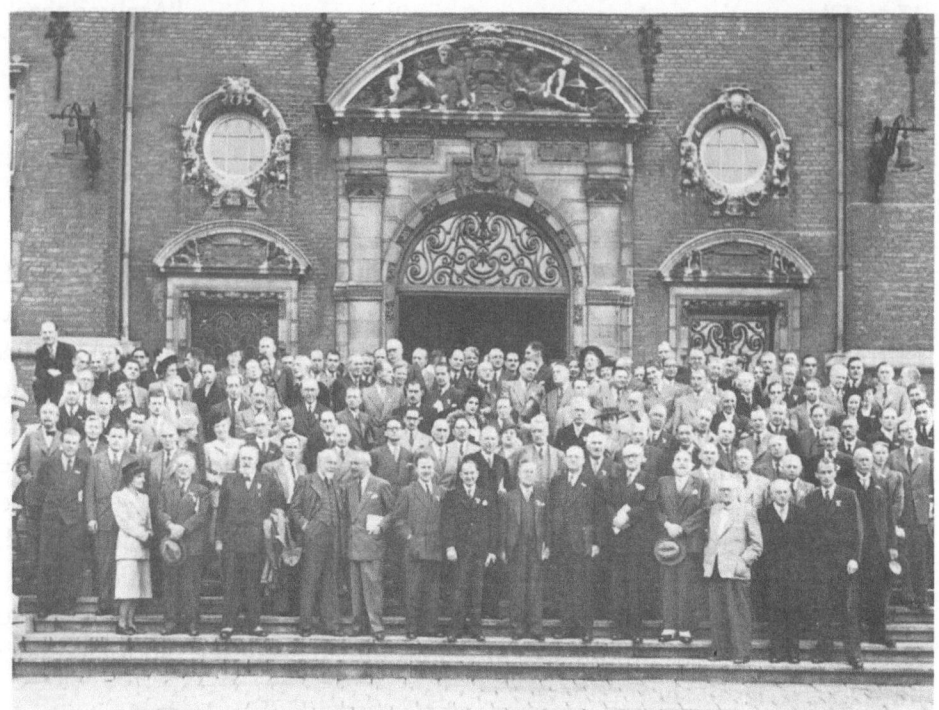

Fig. 13. The attendants of the Amsterdam meeting at the Indisch Instituut

The Instituut had a large and a small lecture hall, and two licensed restaurants. Coffee wa served continuously in the entrance hall, where there was also an exhibition of instruments and books. These diversions were in great demand, for many contributions were delivered in languages whith which few were familiar. In the scientific exhibit, attention was attracted by many excellent instruments for osteosynthesis, which included bone clamps based on the designs of Professor LAMBOTTE who now lives quietly in a suburb of Antwerp, and pursues his hobby of making violins and cellos with superb craftsmanship. The circular saw, designed in Great Britain by Messrs. Desoutter Bros., had been modified by a Belgian firm* in such a way as to act in a longitudinal axis, and the intermittent whine of this instrument was the basic musical note of the congress; it served as a descant to every conversation. Apart from daily scientific sessions at the Instituut, two very

---

* According to suggestions by JEAN DELCHEF and the engineer Fransen of Verviers (communication from JEAN DELCHEF Jr. to the author).

enjoyable evening receptions were held in the Rijksmuseum and the Stedelijke Museum. The galleries were thrown open to members and guests. The Rijksmuseum included not only its own treasures but also the touring Munich collection, and the Stedelijk Museum once again housed its famous collection of VAN GOGHS, so that the receptions were of particular interest.

At the general meeting there was comment and discussion on difficulties which had arisen from the language problem; it was urged by some that contributions should be delivered in French or English, and that lantern slides should include legends in several languages. There was also debate on the constitution of the society and the method by which members and delegates were elected. It was decided that the next congress should be held in Stockholm in 1951, and that Professor SCHERB of Zurich should be the President. The main subjects selected for discussion were "Bone changes in avitaminosis" and "Low back pain". Sir HARRY PLATT (Great Britain) was elected President of the Society and Professor SORREL (France) and Dr. SAN RICART (Spain) were Vice Presidents.

The same proceedings end with a visit to the Anna Clinic of Leyden: The last two days of the conference were devoted to clinical meetings. This writer visited the Anna Clinic* which is famous for the work of MURK JANSEN and is now under the direction of Dr. VAN NES. A large portrait of Sir ROBERT JONES stands in the entrance hall and his signature occupies a place of honour in the visiting book. Dr. VAN NES gave a remarkable demonstration of major surgery on two successive mornings. In the course of four and a half hours operating he performed two cup arthroplasties of the hip, two arthrodeses of the hip, one shortening of the femur with plating and grafting, one spinal fusion with graft, and two capsulectomies of the hip joint. The grace of work was quite remarkable. It was made possible by abandoning the changing of gloves and gown between operations and by using a trained staff to apply all plasters. Throughout the time he was at work, Dr. VAN NES explained his technique in four languages..."

Such was the authentic day-by-day account[19], and to this we must add that there were visits to hospitals in Nijmegen, Utrecht and Laren.

---

* MURK JANSEN wa a powerful fighter in any good cause, and when in 1928 he devoted half his private fortune to the building and equipping of the ANNA KLINIEK, the operating theatre suite on the upper floor was designed on a lavish scale. Its windows could be seen from many parts of the old university of Leiden and were impishly believed by JANSEN to provide a much needed counter-irritant to the professor of surgery as he passed on his bicycle to and from duties at the University Hospital.[14]

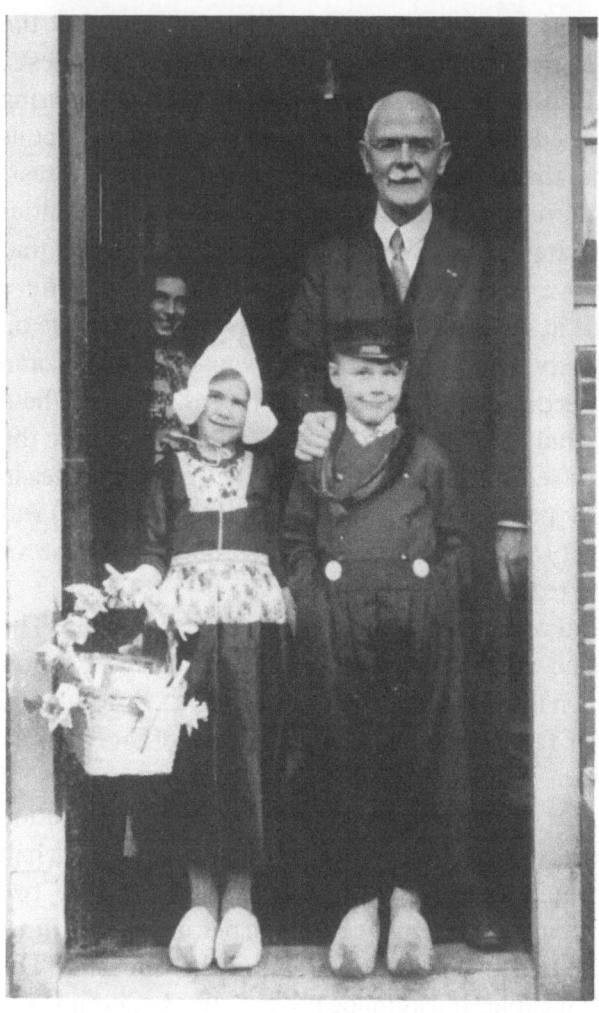

Fig. 14. MURK JANSEN, the dutch giant who inspired the Amsterdam meeting

This first really large-scale post-war congress pointed up a major difficulty: the language problem. And the way in which the problem was tackled is further proof of the vitality of S.I.C.O.T. The very next of this Amsterdam congress, the Editor of the journal *Bone and Surgery* remarked[20]: "As a social occasion the meeting was so great a success as to warrant the belief that such gatherings are justified if for no other reason than *the surgeons of many countries may meet and get to know each other.*"*

---

* Author's underlining.

54

One day there were forty-two papers, each with a ten minute limit. One correspondent writes "Many speakers had much more than twenty minutes' material to present within ten minute limit and they were determined to beat the red light. They spoke at three times the normal rate and few of us understood a word. If these meetings are to be regarded as no more than social occasions we must apply ourselves to the language problem, which has been solved at international political conferences and can surely be solved at international scientific meetings."

In fact S.I.C.O.T. did solve the problem; Englisch was progressively adopted as the common language, as spoken language and eventually as the language of publication (International Committee of Budapest, October 1974).* The leaders of S.I.C.O.T. also wisely set up the "Review Lectures" and "Instructional Courses", which further alleviated the problem. If S.I.C.O.T. was able to get off on a good footing in this difficult post-war period it was to a large extent due to the fine qualities of our Dutch colleagues.

A final word on the social events. On Monday 13 September, following the inaugural session, the President of the Congress and Mrs. MEYERDING gave a reception in the hall of the Indisch Instituut. The day ended in the galleries of the Rijksmuseum[21] where the congress participants and their families were the guests of the Dutch government. On Wednesday 15 September, the municipality of Amsterdam received the participants at the Stedelijk Museum[22], where there was a retrospective of Van Gogh and the visitors were able to feast their eyes on the marvellous colours. The congress closed with a banquet at which there were of course many speeches, and culminated in the conferring of diplomas. One small detail: A commemorative medal had been struck, but we should point out that it mentions Sir ROBERT JONES among the founders, which as we have seen is historically inaccurate. A further point of interest was the visit to the Ijsselmeer or Zuyderzee, as it was formerly known, which was reclaimed by the Dutch with their indefatigable genius.

---

* 80% English, 20% French, to be precise.

Fourth Congress: Amsterdam 13–18 September 1948

Officers of the Meeting

President: HENRY W. MEYERDING
Vice President: CORNELIS SCHAAP
Secretary: J. D. MULDER

Reports

1. *"Le traitement des arthrites déformantes de la hanche"*
   (Treatment of coxarthritis)
   PAUL MATHIEU and PAUL PADOVANI
   JAN ZAHRADNICEK
   ELOI HUBERT LA CHAPELLE
   JEAN DELCHEF
   GUNNAR WIBERG
   MARIUS N. SMITH PETERSEN

2. *"Les traumatismes fermés du rachis"*
   (Closed injuries of the spine)
   E. A. NICOLL
   LORENZ BOEHLER
   CARLO PAIS
   C. ELKINS and HENRY W. MEYERDING
   RAMON SAN RICART

Free Papers: 36

Officers of the Society

President: LOUIS OMBREDANNE
Vice Presidents: RAMON SAN RICART
                   Sir HARRY PLATT
Secretary General: JEAN DELCHEF
Treasurer: CHARLES PARISEL

56

Stockholm, 21–25 May 1951[23]

A quite exceptional privilege was accorded to this fifth S.I.C.O.T. congress: His Majesty GUSTAVE VI ADOLPHE of Sweden attended the inaugural session. It was the first time that a head of state had honoured our society with his presence.

This inaugural session took place on 21 May at 11 a.m. in the Great Concert Hall of the Palace of Stockholm. Present were representatives of the government, of the municipal council of Stockholm, and numerous Swedish medical authorities. There were about 400 participants, half of whom were members of S.I.C.O.T. The National Anthem was played as the king entered, after which there several speeches, interspersed with some very pleasant music.

HENNING WALDENSTRÖM, Honorary President of the Congress, gave the first address, thanking His Majesty King GUSTAVE VI ADOLPHE, the authorities and the organisers, and welcoming the participants. The programme of social events was also announced. STEN FRIBERG gave an address on behalf of RICHARD SCHERB*, President of the Congress, which clearly and judiciously gave an account of the current state of our special field and its future prospects. Sir HARRY PLATT, President of S.I.C.O.T., thanked the Swedish hosts on behalf of all the participants.

According to tradition, the scientific programme entailed two reports, the first on "Advitaminosis and bone diseases" and the second on "Low back pain and sciatic pain". It should be noted that the leaders of S.I.C.O.T., ever conscious of the society's role in the progress of orthopaedic surgery, were setting up one of the first important beacons in Europe on the second of these subjects. It was in 1933 that JOSEPH BARR published the first work on this nosological entity, differentiating it from the general (and vast) category of low back pain. For this reason, and also because of its fundamental importance, the question was in fact broached first. There were 34 contributions to the discussion, which shows how much interest the question aroused. The free papers dealt, among other matters, with the relatively new questions of the use of radio isotopes and arthroscopy. There was further

* Who had to remain in Switzerland due to illness.

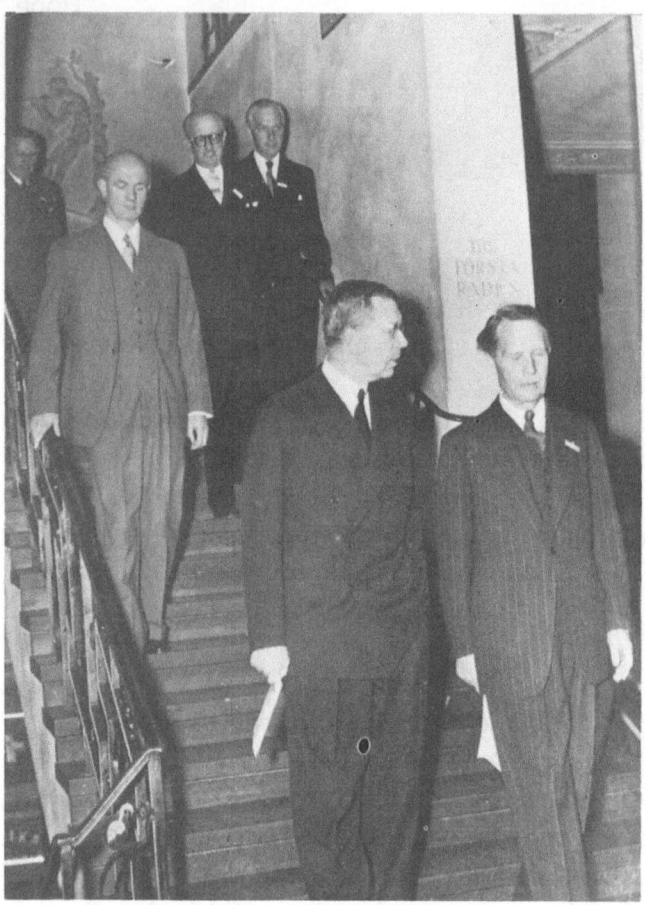

Fig. 15. H. M. KING GUSTAV VI ADOLPH and the hosts: WALDENSTRÖM, STEN FRIBERG, JEAN DELCHEF, HARALD NILSONNE and Sir HARRY PLATT

demonstration of the ever-increasing interest in the society in the admission of more countries: India, Japan and Portugal. Curiously enough China had also been admitted, but only through a representative living in New York. At the same time the first Japanese member was admitted, and in honour of our hosts at the anniversary congress I would like to mention him by name: Mr. MIKI ISAHARU. The social events were once again an opportunity to show the friendship and fraternisation among members of the association.

There were many delights for the members and their families visiting one of the most beautiful capital cities of the world populated by the most hospitable and courteous peoples. Nearly all had at least one private invitation and were able to witness the artistic provision of food, drink and

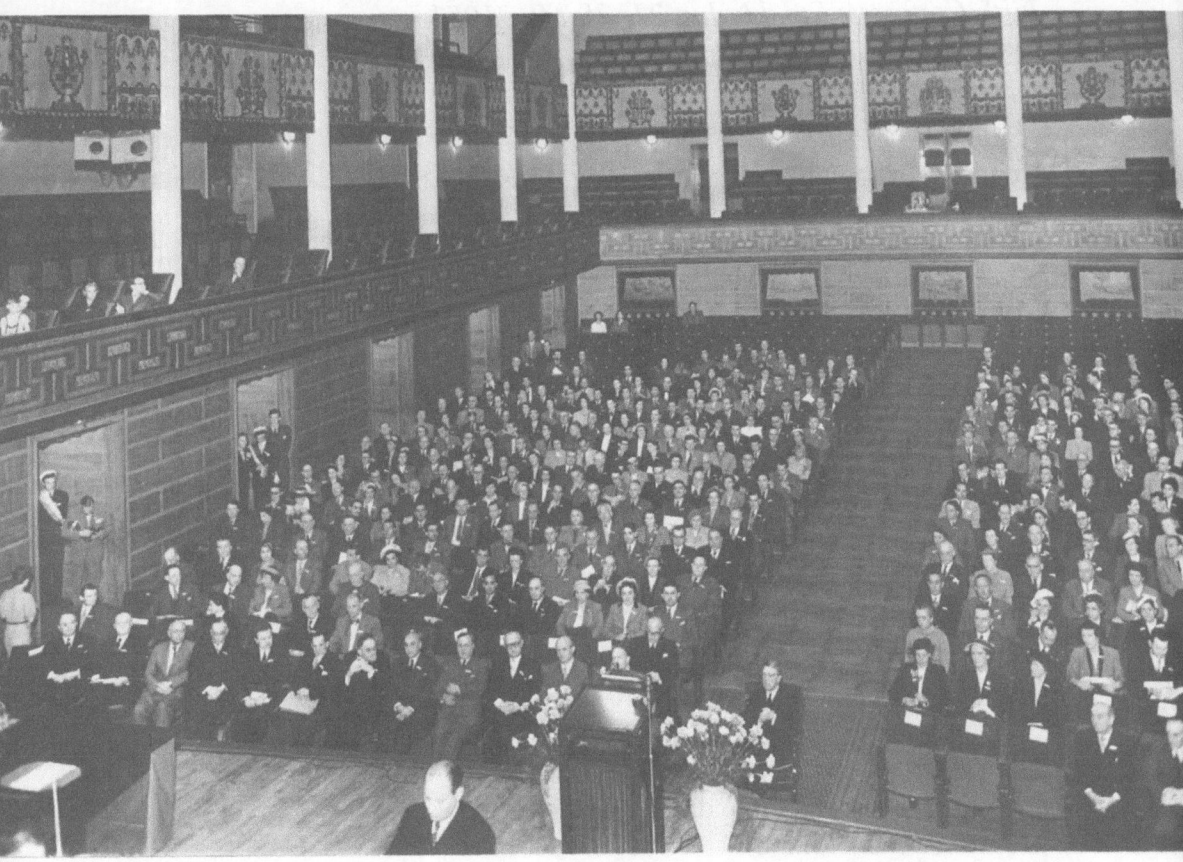

Fig. 16. H. M. KING GUSTAV VI ADOLPH and the participants of the Stockholm meeting

entertainment for large numbers in small homes. Official invitations included a soirée at the National Museum, where it was possible to enjoy a concert by the Stockholm Chamber Orchestra and see many works by the old masters and others. Perhaps the most delightful entertainment was first a City reception in the beautiful Town Hall and thence by water to the Palace of Drottningholm[25], where supper (described in a masterpiece of understatement as a "picnic") was taken in the foyer of the eighteenth-century State Theater, in which afterwards members were enchanted by ballet and music of the eighteenth century given by members of the ballet and artists of the Royal Opera. The week finished with a banquet for some four hundred guests at the Grand Hotel Royal where diversions included students' songs and dancing. It would be wrong to close this summary of the Congress without mentioning the excellence of the organisation, which was, if possible, as outstanding as the hospitality.[23,24]

Fifth Congress: Stockholm, 21–25 May 1951

Officers of the Meeting

Honorary President*: HENNING WALDENSTRÖM
President: RICHARD SCHERB
Vice President: STEN FRIBERG
Secretary: ANDERS KARLEN
Treasurer: HARALD NILSONNE

Reports

1. *Lombosciatalgie, résultats du traitement*
   (Low back pain and sciatic pain; results of treatment)
   JOSEPH BARR
   R. H. YOUNG
   LOUIS POUYANNE
   Discussion: 36 speakers

2. *Avitaminose et ostéopathie***
   (Avitaminosis and bone diseases)
   RAFAELE ZANOLI

Free Papers: 46

Officers of the Society

Honorary President*: LOUIS OMBREDANNE
President: Sir HARRY PLATT
Vice Presidents: RAMON SAN RICART
ETIENNE SORREL
Secretary General: JEAN DELCHEF
Treasurer: CHARLES PARISEL

---

* Honorary President is not exactly "Président d'Honneur", but we cannot find a better translation.
** This Report was in fact the first one, but because of the importance of low back pain it was decided to start with the second report.

Bern, 30 August–3 September 1954[25]

To within a few days, the sixth congress coincided with the 25th anniversary of the founding of the society. This stage is what is commonly known as 'adulthood', and in many families – which is how JEAN DELCHEF used to talk of his beloved S.I.C.O.T.[28] – the occasion is marked by the giving of a present, a jewel. And this in fact is what happened. On Tuesday 31 August, BRYAN MCFARLAND, who at that time was President of the British Orthopaedic Association, presented on behalf of the English members of the society[27, p. 698] a badge of office to be worn by the presidents of S.I.C.O.T. The President, Sir HARRY PLATT, accepted it, and passed it on forthwith to ETIENNE SORREL, president of the Bern congress. Here is an excerpt from the address he gave, which is characterises the affection which united all the members: *"Quand nous nous reverrons, d'ici trois ans, notre Société sera déjà entrée dans son deuxième quart de siècle, ayant toujours eu pour but d'encourager l'esprit d'entente et l'amitié entre les chirurgiens orthopédistes du monde entier."** (When we meet again in three years' time, our society will already have entered into its second quarter century, having always had as its aim the fostering of a spirit of understanding and friendship among the orthopaedic surgeons of the whole world.)

As we can see throughout the history of S.I.C.O.T., friendship and understanding have not failed to be a constant *leitmotiv*.

Unfortunately adulthood is also the time when we begin to suffer the passing on of the older members of the family. Our association was by no means exempt from this law of nature; and of the original 21 there were now only 13. Since 1929 the following had died: MACHARD († 1931), BAER († 1931), MURK JANSEN († 1931), HAGLUND († 1934), PUTTI († 1940), ALBEE († 1945), MAFFEI († 1945) and GALEAZZI († 1952). But once more the flow of life asserted itself, ensuring the continuation of our work and the passing on of the torch: 42 countries were represented and the society now had 528 members.

Adulthood also brings new problems in its wake, about which the older and wiser may of course be consulted; but enquiries can also be made outside the immediate community to ensure that the best possible advice has been

---

* Spoken in French by Sir HARRY.

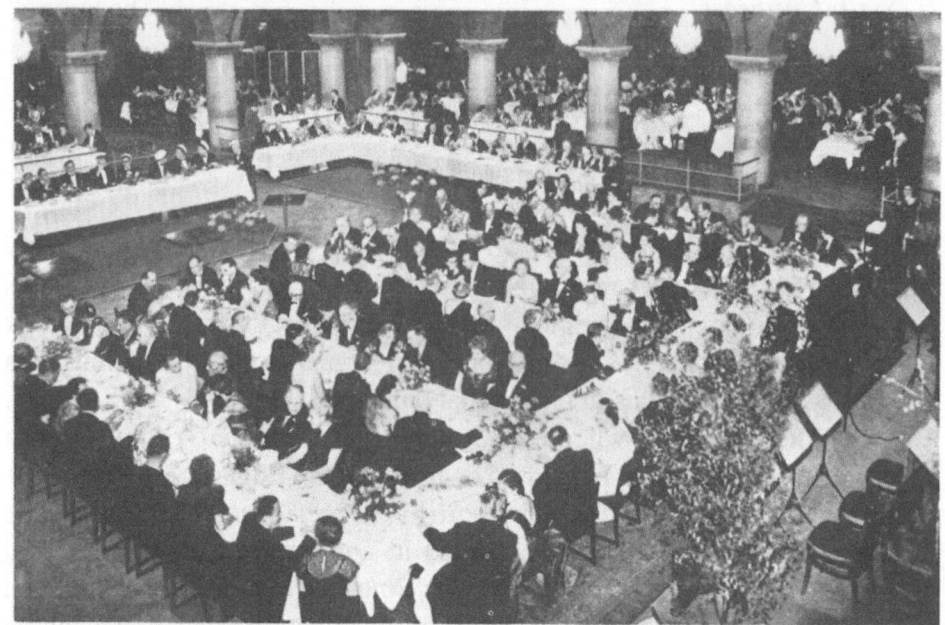

Fig. 17. The closing banquet in the Vintertradgärden at the Grand Hotel Royal

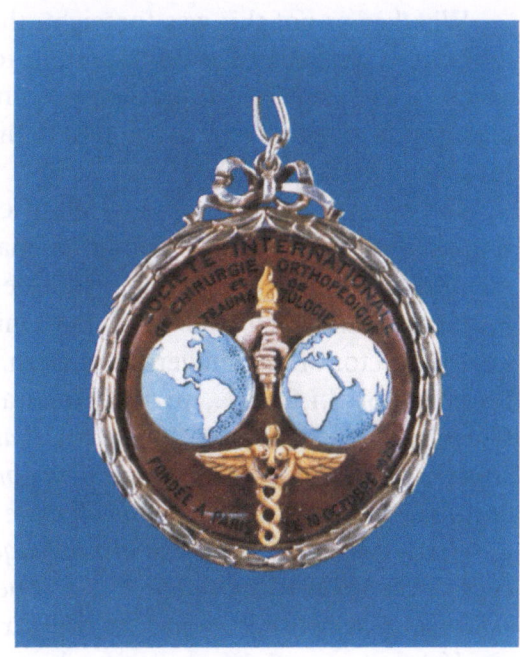

Fig. 18. The badge of office presented to the President of the society by the British Members

obtained and all possible resources examined. This is what S.I.C.O.T. was to do. Confronted with growing pains and – it is no secret – with financial problems – *(nil novi sub sole!)* our leaders consulted ... and obtained financial aid from the Conseil des Organisations Internationales des Sciences Médicales, C.I.O.M.S.* On this occasion the role of the big international congresses was defined, with particular reference to the long-windedness which often wastes so much time: *"Les grands Congrès Internationaux ne devraient avoir qu'un but: enseigner. Les Congrès devraient faire connaître les progrès les plus récents de la Médecine à un auditoire, aussi nombreux, aussi jeune et aussi international que possible. En conséquence, une place beaucoup moins importante devrait être consacrée à la discussion."* (The big international congresses should have one aim only: to teach. The congress should make known the most recent progress in medicine to an auditorium as full, as young and as international as possible. Therefore far less weight should be given to discussion.)

---

* Initials of Council for International Organizations of Medical Sciences.

Whether or not this was foresight, the organisers of this sixth congress introduced the idea of the symposium for the first time, and no less than seven symposia were arranged. It was an arrangement which proved to be most productive and of great benefit to the participants, and was retained in future congresses.[26, p. 108]

The opening session was particularly ceremonious, reflecting the age-old traditions of Switzerland. Among the many personages present we should mention the following by name: Monsieur P. ETTER, Federal Councillor; Professor ALDER, Pro-rector of the University of Bern; and Professor P. LIVER, Rector of the University of Bern, who admitted Sir HARRY PLATT, President of S.I.C.O.T., to the Honorary Doctorate in Medicine of the University[27, p. 685], saying: *"Sir Harry Platt, élève remarquable de Sir Robert Jones, de Manchester, a non seulement poursuivi l'oeuvre de son maître, mais encore lui a donné un essor considérable en prenant une parte éminente au développement de la chirurgie orthopédique anglo-saxonne. Celle-ci, grâce à cette collaboration importante, est devenue un édifice imposant dont la valeur est universellement reconnue. Ses travaux chirurgicaux traitent spécialement des lésions traumatiques des nerfs, des paralysies, des affections articulaires congénitales et acquises, des maladies des os. Ils sont ceux d'un maître qui s'est*

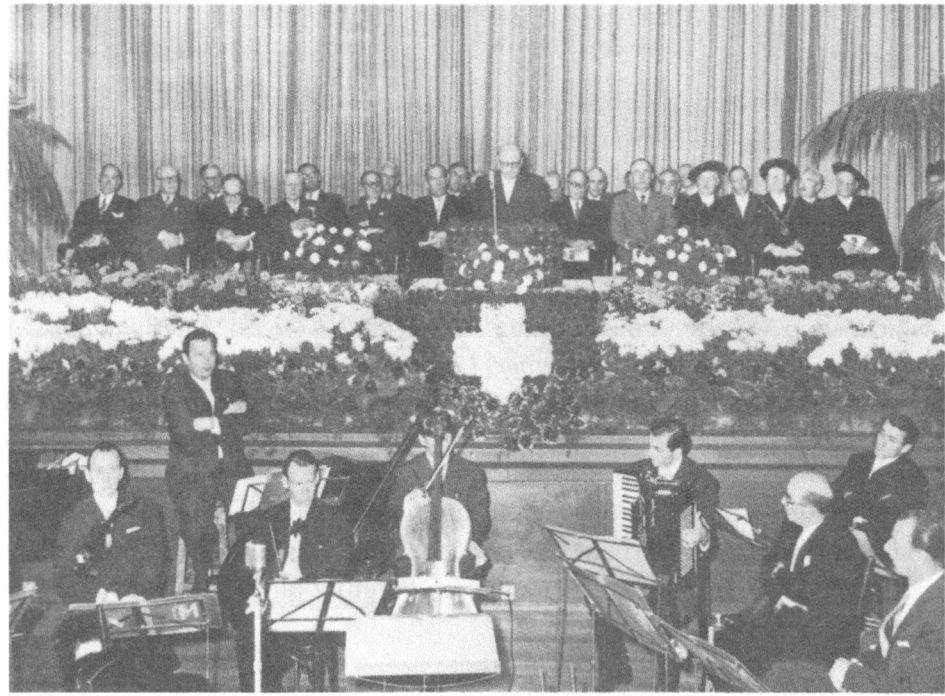

Fig. 19. The opening ceremony at the Kursaal in Bern

révélé aussi un parfait organisateur. Son oeuvre médico-sociale est des plus importantes. Il a pris une part active au développement de la Médecine tant sur le plan biologique que social, développement indispensable dans un état moderne."[27] (Sir Harry Platt, that most remarkable pupil of Sir Robert Jones of Manchester, not only continued the work of his mentor but also gave it considerable impetus by taking an eminent part in the development of Anglo-Saxon orthopaedic surgery, which thanks to him has grown to imposing proportions, and its value is universally recognised. Sir Harry's surgical work deals primarily with traumatic lesions of the nerves, paralysis, articular disorders, both congenital and acquired, and bone diseases. It is the work of a master who has also shown himself to be a perfect organiser. His medico-social work is of particular importance. He has played an active part in the development of medicine on both the biological and the social plane, the latter being a vital development in present-day society.)

Many speeches were made, and for the sake of completeness we should mention those of MARCEL DUBOIS, the organising spirit behind the congress; of Monsieur ETTER, the Federal Councillor; of RICHARD SCHERB*, Honorary President of the Congress, read by ETIENNE SORREL; and finally of ETIENNE SORREL himself, in his capacity as President of the Congress: *"De l'entité que constitue la Chirurgie osseuse telle que la comprenaient les fondateurs de la Société Internationale de Chirurgie Orthopédique lors de sa création le 10 octobre 1929."* (The entity constituted by Bone Surgery as understood by the founders of S.I.C.O. at the time of its foundation in October 1929.) It is a fine tribute to the vision of our founders and a plea for continuing progress and untiring research in our special field.

The following day the scientific session commenced, as no one will be surprised to hear that they ran with clockwork precision from start to finish. A further innovation was added along with the symposia; an opportunity for the participants to learn the maximum amount possible without wasting any time. On the programme there were various visits to Swiss hospitals: Basle, Bern/Macolin, Geneva, Lausanne/Leysin and Zurich; this particular improvement was dubbed 'satellite meetings', and the credit for the idea is certainly due to the organisers of the Bern congress. Two exhibitions, one scientific and one historical, provided further opportunities for the truly avid to satisfy their thirst for knowledge.

---

* Already ill in 1951 and unable to preside over the Stockholm congress, as we have seen, RICHARD SCHERB was still bedridden; he died the following year.

65

The Swiss were perfect hosts, offering all their country's resources to enable everyone to return home with the pleasantest of memories. The Bernese countryside, the local cuisine, the folk choruses, dances, songs and traditional costumes, were all thoroughly enchanting. The banquet, too, had the Swiss touch; it was simple, friendly and pleasant. Then for the more athletic participants, a climb up the Jungfraujoch enabled them to stretch their legs and dispel their surplus energy. A concert of religious music in the cathedral delighted the music lovers with its austere beauty. Before we leave the sixth congress we should mention an important change in the composition of the committee. Having fulfilled the role of secretary for 25 years, JEAN DELCHEF found himself called upon to take on the presidency of the society. Many of us had the privilege of knowing him; but even having been among those close to him towards the end of his life, I do not know what his feelings were at this moment. Pride, certainly, and also awareness of the honour bestowed upon him; but perhaps also a certain sadness, a contraction of the heart – as when one of your children marries and you feel a slight sense of loss. Having devoted 25 years to bringing up the society, having cradled it in his arms through circumstances that were often far from easy, he must have had mixed feelings; but in his heart, we may be sure, his greatest wish to serve S.I.C.O.T.

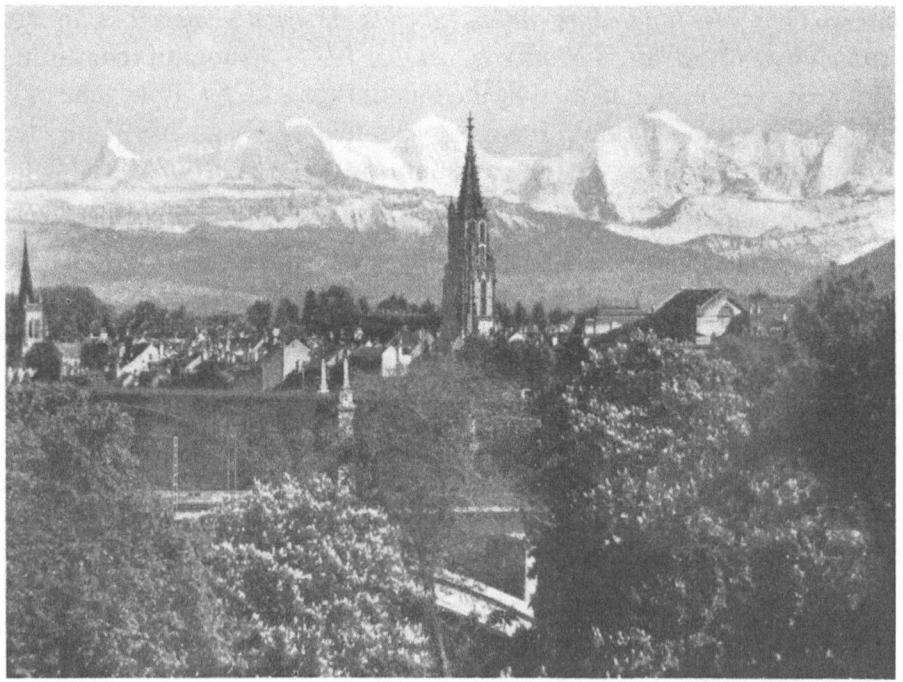

Fig. 20. The peaks surrounding Bern, the place of the sixth meeting, another peak for S.I.C.O.T.

Sixth Congress: Bern, 30 August to 3 September 1954

Officers of the Congress

Honorary President: RICHARD SCHERB
President: ETIENNE SORREL
Vice President: MARCEL DUBOIS
Secretary General: MAX RENÉ FRANCILLON
CHARLES SCHOLDER
Treasurer: HANS DEBRUNNER

Reports

1. *Traitement de la scoliose*
   (Treatment of scoliosis)
   BRYAN MCFARLAND
   J. I. P. JAMES
   OSKAR A. STRACKER
   F. G. ALLAN
   Discussion: 22 speakers

2. *La chirurgie de la main*
   (Surgery of the hand)
   ROBERT MERLE D' AUBIGNÉ
   JORG BOEHLER
   JEAN GOSSET
   MICHAEL MASON and JOHN BELL
   GUY PULVERTAFT
   RAOUL TUBIANA
   Discussion: 12 speakers

Free Papers: 62

Symposia

Problèmes de chirurgie orthopédique et de traumatologie en gérontologie (Orthopaedic surgery and traumatology in elderly people)
Les bases physiologiques de l'effort maxima dans les sports (Basic physiology of the maximum effort in sport)
Coxarthrose (Arthritis of the hip)
Physiopathologie des fractures (Physiopathology of fractures)
La tuberculose osteo-articulaire (Tuberculosis of the joints)
La dégénérescence musculaire et son traitement (Muscle atrophy and its treatment)
Physiologie et pathologie de la locomotion (Motion: physiology and pathology)
Les bases légales de la médecine des accidents en Suisse (Forensic medicine of injuries in Switzerland)
Anatomie et pathologie du muscle (Anatomy and pathology of muscle)

Officer of the Society

Honorary President: LOUIS OMBREDANNE
President: Sir HARRY PLATT
Vice Presidents: ETIENNE SORREL
JOSÉ VALLS
Secretary General: JEAN DELCHEF
Treasurer: CHARLES PARISEL

68

Barcelona, 16–21 September 1957[29]

On 3 March 1492 three graceful sailing ships, the *Pinta*, the *Nina* and the *Santa Maria*, left the little port of Palos, South West Spain, in the province of Huelva. The admiral in command was none other than CHRISTOPHER COLUMBUS (1451–1506) who, as is well known, was to discover the New World. On his return in March 1493, he was received in triumph by the monarchs, FERDINAND V of Aragon (1452–1516) and ISABELLE of Castille (1474–1504) at Barcelona. Four and a half centuries later another triumphal reception awaited the orthopaedic surgeons of the world; and Columbus's three sailing ships would not have been sufficient to carry all the participants in this seventh S.I.C.O.T. congress. The palace of Montjuich[31] was to be the scene of their activities for five days.

The inaugural session took place on Monday 16 September at 4 p.m. On the platform numerous military, civic, academic and religious personages were grouped around the Captain General of the 4th Military Region, PABLO MARTIN ALONSO, and JEAN DELCHEF, who, having so often assisted the president in office, was presiding for the first time himself. There were a great many speeches, as befits the land of Cervantes. JOSÉ M. VILLARDEL, secretary of the congress, welcomed the participants, who with

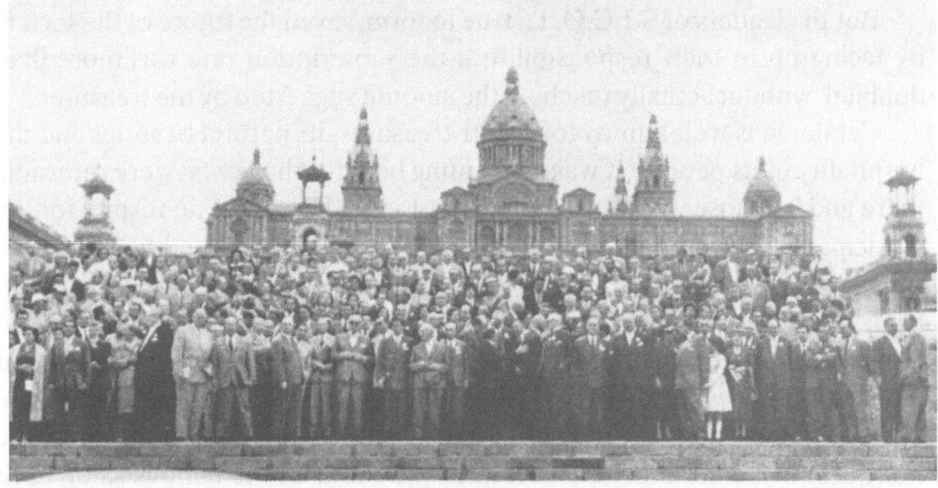

Fig. 21. The participants of the seventh meeting in front of the Palace of Montjuich, Barcelona

their families numbered more than a thousand, and gave a vote of thanks to the autorities. The President, JEAN DELCHEF, followed him by greeting all the authorities individually. JOSÉ VALLS, President of the congress and at the same time Vice President of the Society, followed with an address on the state of orthopaedic surgery and traumatology in the Spanish-speaking countries of South America, in honour of the Spanish hosts. The wealth of historical detail provided by "Pepe" Valls is a source of very valuable information to the historian. El Señor GARCIA ORCOYEN, Director General of Health, and el Señor F. ACEDO COLUNGA, Civil Governor, extended a welcome to the participants on behalf of the Catalan authorities.

The scientific work began the next day, and by all accounts it was up to the usual standards. The idea of the symposium, first adopted in Bern, was retained, but at the same time the number was reduced to three, which were consequently better attended. Another new aspect was the reduction of the number of free papers by a selection committee, which later became a programme committee – one of the principal means by which the standard of future congresses was to be raised.

At the general assembly, two new countries were admitted: Ecuador and Thailand. ANTOINE BAILLEUX, a faithful disciple of JEAN DELCHEF, had succeeded the latter as Secretary General, to which post he in his turn became devoted. For the sake of historical completeness which should mention that the treasurer, JOSEPH CORNET, who had also just taken up office, had the painful task of reporting a "debit" due to the usual reasons (both then and nowadays), namely the costs of printing and the postal charges.

But the leaders of S.I.C.O.T., true to form, saved the future of the society by facing up to their responsibilities; the subscription rate was more than doubled, without actually reaching the amount suggested by the treasurer...

Catalonia is well known for its art treasures, its natural beauties and the hospitality of its people. It was enchanting both for those who were returning there and for those who were on their first visit. There was no respite for the participants (but no one was complaining), who were invited to partake of some splendid festivities every evening. Hardly had the inaugural session been brought to a close than the entire congress met up in the "Barrio Gotico" to wander at will in a maze of picturesque streets, lined with ancient monuments and watched over by the cathedral. These indefatigable people "began" the evening at the Palace of the Permanent Deputation, where the Marquess of Castel-Florite entertained his guests in the famous salon of St George. The evening continued at the "El Cortijo" restaurant, with classic Iberian dancing which went on late into the night.[32]

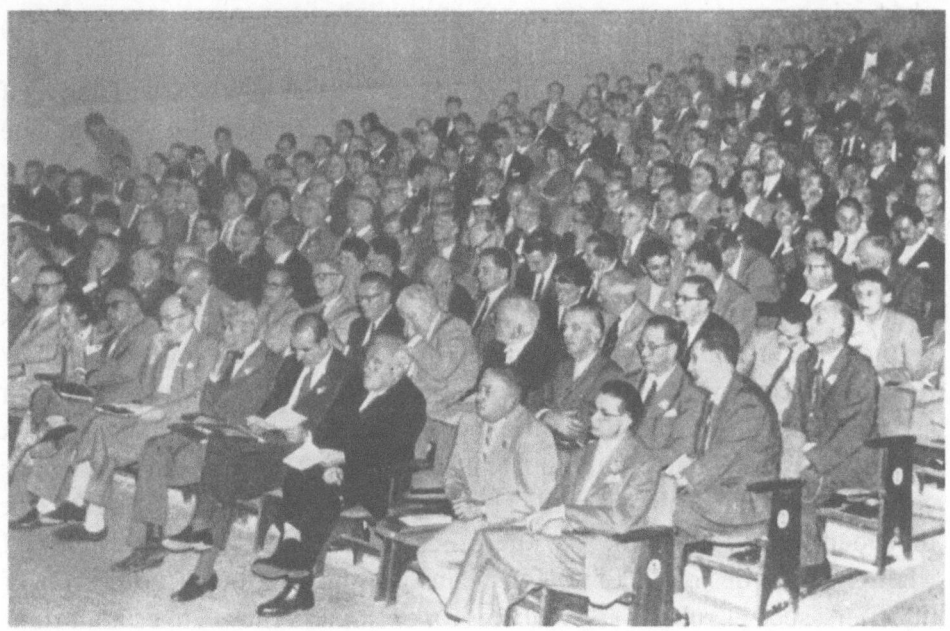

Fig. 22. The audience at the Barcelona meeting

Equally magnificent was the reception the next day, Tuesday 17 September, courtesy of the Alcalde of Barcelona, Señor Don JOSÉ MARIA DE PORCIOLES COLOMER, at the town hall. Treasures of art and architecture met the eager eyes of the participants at every turn. The following day, it was time for an open-air festival of Catalan dances and music. Spain of course means bullfights, and the following evening, Thursday 19 September, quite a few of the participants of the congress discovered to their delight that they were "aficionados". The culmination of the congress was the banquet on Friday 20 September, which was also held in the splendid Palace of Montjuich, where the participants cordially took leave of one another after a most memorable week.

To end on a rather sad note: The 21 were now reduced to 10. JEAN DELCHEF had indeed presided over these revels, but it was the only time Destiny was to allow him this pleasure and this honour.*

---

* The 'Proceedings' also give notice of the deeply felt loss of the master of all, LOUIS OMBREDANNE, the year before the Barcelona congress. His spirit, so warmly evoked in the death announcement, hovered over all those present.

Addendum

This congress at Barcelona was in a manner of speaking the second pang of conscience on the part of S.I.C.O.T. as regards its responsibility to medicine on a worldwide scale – a kind of "extroversion", if we may put it thus. We saw how relations were established in Bern with C.I.O.M.S.; one of the resolutions passed by the Barcelona congress, or more precisely by the general assembly, ran thus: In view of the serious problem presented by congenital deformities and the obscurity of their causation, the Congress recommended that its members should take the following action in their respective countries: 1) to endeavour to establish research units in appropriate centers in collaboration with other interested workers, such as obstetricians, paediatricians and embryologists; 2) to point out to their governments the social and medical importance of the problem, and to seek the financial aid necessary for the prosecution of research; 3) when and where it seems desirable, to ask for the institution of statutory notification of disorders, such as rubella and diabetes for example, believed to be important in the etiology of congenital disorders.

Seventh Congress: Barcelona, 16–21 September 1957

Officers of the Meeting

President: JOSÉ VALLS
Vice President: MANUEL BASTOS ANSART
Secretary: JOSÉ VILLARDEL
Treasurer: ANGEL SANTOS PALAZZI

Reports

1. *Le traitement des articulations ballantes*
   (Treatment of flail joints)
   GEORG HOHMANN
   MANUEL BASTOS ANSART
   OSCAR SCAGLIETTI and GIORGIO FINESCHI
   Discussion: 7 speakers

2. *L'influence de la croissance sur les sequelles des traumatismes chez l'enfant*
   (Influence of growth on the sequelae of injuries in childhood)
   JOSÉ TRUETA
   PAUL-LOUIS CHIGOT
   WALTER P. BLOUNT
   BRYAN MCFARLAND
Discussion: 13 speakers

Free Papers: 30

3. *Symposia*
Les tumeurs à cellules géantes et leur traitment (Giant cell tumours and their treatment)
Le traitement chirurgical de l'arthrose de la hanche excepté l'arthroplastie (Surgical treatment of coxarthritis, except arthroplasty)
Les causes et la prévention des malformations congénitales du rachis et des membres (Causes and preventive treatment of congenital malformations of the spine and limbs)

Officers of the Society

President: JEAN DELCHEF
Vice Presidents: JOSÉ VALLS
                         JOSEPH TRUETA
Secretary General: ANTOINE BAILLEUX
Treasurer: CHARLES PARISEL

New York, 4–9 September 1960[33]

The outstanding feature of this congress was, in my view, the hospitality –
American style, if I may put it thus. Scanning the programme, one constantly
finds: reception and cocktail party, special hospitality evening, free events,
etc.... There is nothing surprising in this; the United States in general and
New York in particular are renowned for one essential characteristic: the
melting pot, of which hospitality is the most agreeable result. Feeling at ease,
and making sure one's guests feel at ease, is a speciality of the American
people.

In several ways the New York congress was symbolic. First of all it was the
first time that S.I.C.O.T. had held its congress outside 'good old Europe',
becoming aware of its truly international responsibilities. Secondly, the pang
of conscience felt in Bern (leading to the intervention of C.I.O.M.S.) and in
Barcelona (with the motion on malformations) about the responsibility of
the society in teaching, research and education had not abated: The
symposium, which was unique in the importance of its subject, was about
*"L'Enseignement de la chirurgie orthopédique et de la traumatologie et
l'organisation des services dans les hôpitaux"* (Teaching and training in
orthopaedic surgery and traumatology and the organization of hospital
services). The personalities and nationalities both of the moderators and of
the participants in the subsequent discussion were a further symbol of the
international role of the society.

Thirdly, whether by good fortune or deliberate choice, the personality of
the president, JOSEPH TRUETA, reflected these international aspects, while
he was also one of the most loyal and enthusiastic members of S.I.C.O.T. He
was not unaware of this himself, and his inaugural speech is most
characteristic in this respect. Here are the main passages from it, shot
through with his special brand of humour which is neither exactly Catalan nor
exactly English:

"It is customary because it is unavoidable to open a Presidential Address
with words of recognition for the honour of having been elected to the
Presidency ... Moreover two circumstances gave particular significance to
my election ... The first was that your decision to elect me to the presidency
took place in Barcelona, the place of my birth. The second was that with your
choice you dissipated any doubts I could have as to the wisdom of my decision

to leave Catalonia for England at the end of the war in Spain. If I have gained so much of your affection, my exile has not been, as on so many occasions, a sterilising experience. On looking back after twenty years of British life, I cannot but be grateful to God for the privilege offered to me to live with my wife and children in the country where human untolerance is at its lowest. I sincerely believe that in electing me you kindly overlooked my personal characteristics and achievements, and considered instead the peculiarity of my Fate which caused the division of may adult life into two equal parts, the first as Catalan-Spaniard – and thus Latin – and the second as a British subject – thus Anglo-saxon."

Trueta went on by reviewing[34]

"... the state of orthopaedics in general. At the time of the first Congress, held in Paris in 1930, rickets, tuberculosis, poliomyelitis accounted for the vast majority of cripples. These diseases were no longer of national importance. But in spite of this, there was no reduction of orthopaedic work. The surgery of injuries was increasing enormously, and degenerative disease was more frequent because people lived longer. More time is now devoted to research."

There was new evidence of the extension of the role of S.I.C.O.T. Shortly before the congress, a symposium was organised at Princeton under the patronage of S.I.C.O.T., by the C.I.O.M.S. under the auspices of the World Health Organisation and UNESCO.

As far as the social events were concerned, the European-style receptions and festivities 'en masse' were, if I may say so, reduced to a reasonable level, since the mores of hospitalitiy in America in general, and in New York in particular, favour smaller receptions of a more personal nature. Nonetheless there were two occasions on which large numbers of the participants and their families gathered together for festivities. One of the highlights of the entertainments was a mini-cruise on the Hudson River around Manhattan, which allowed everyone to see for themselves the legendary splendour of New York City. Another 'hit' was a performance of "My Fair Lady" to which the participants were invited.[35]

In true American style, all the social events were held in the numerous rooms of one building, the Hotel Astor.[36] The Grand Ballroom was the perfect setting for the closing banquet and ball; and the toasts were proposed by HAROLD SOFIELD, PHILIP D. WILSON, Sir HARRY PLATT and JOSEPH TRUETA. One sad shadow was cast over the proceedings: to everyone's deep regret, the president, JEAN DELCHEF, much against his will was too ill to attend, and was unable to propose the final toast. He was never again to see his friends at S.I.C.O.T.

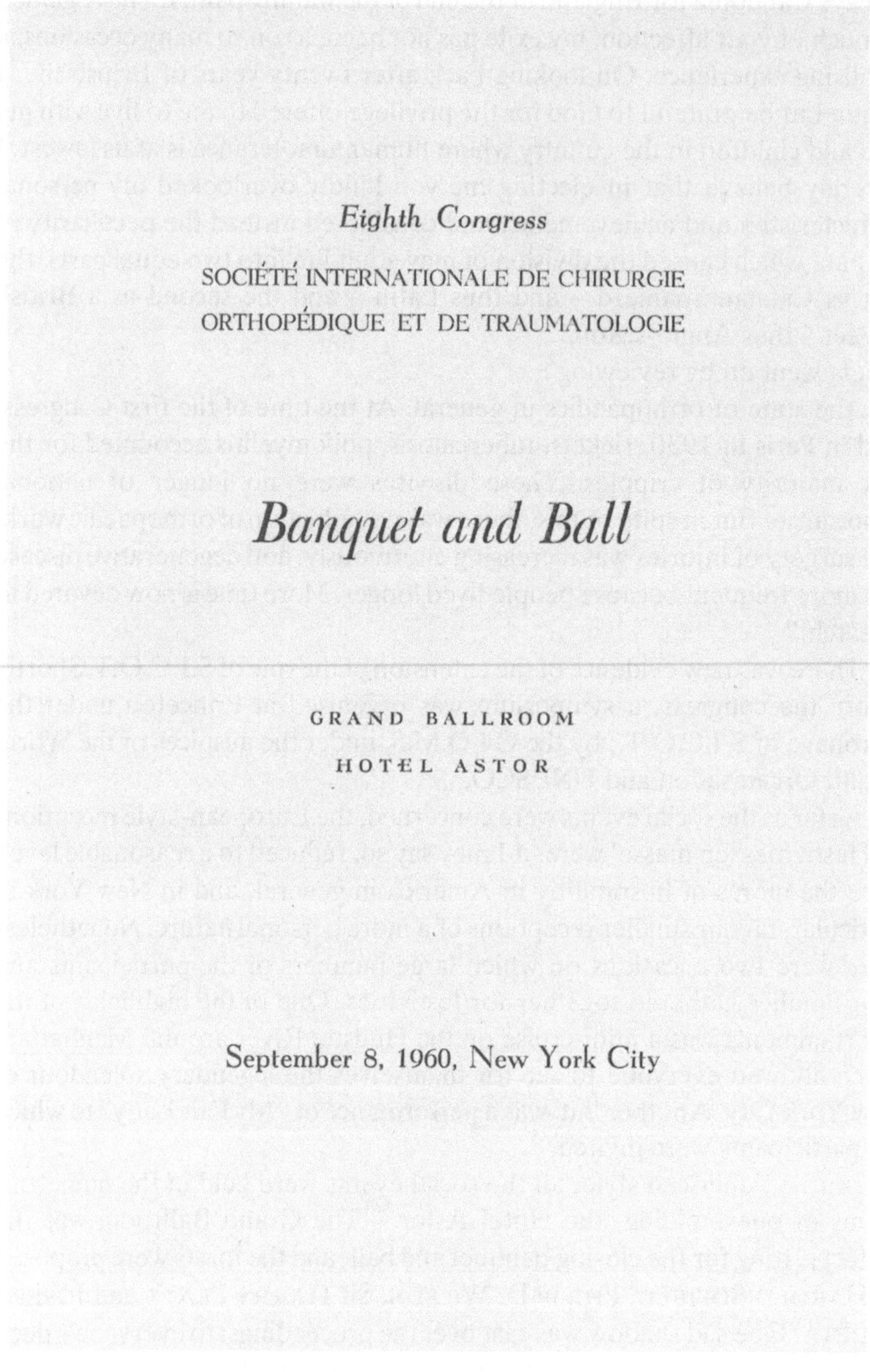

Eighth Congress

SOCIÉTÉ INTERNATIONALE DE CHIRURGIE

ORTHOPÉDIQUE ET DE TRAUMATOLOGIE

Banquet and Ball

GRAND BALLROOM

HOTEL ASTOR

September 8, 1960, New York City

Fig. 23. The Souvenir menu sent from New York to JEAN DELCHEF signed by his friends (see Fig. 24)

Eighth Congress: New York, 4–10 September 1960

Officers of the Meeting

President: JOSEPH TRUETA
Vice President: PHILIP D. WILSON
Secretary: LEE RAMSAY STRAUB
Treasurer: MATHER CLEVELAND

Reports
1. *La dysplasie congénitale de la hanche* (Congenital dysplasia of the hip)
   BRYAN MCFARLAND
   IAN ALVIK
   OSCAR SCAGLIETTI
   BRUNO CALANDRIELLO
   MARCO ORTOLANI
   Discussion: 28 speakers

2. *L'ostéogenèse dans ses rapports avec les retards de consolidation et les pseudoarthroses des os longs* (The study of osteogenesis and its relation to delayed union and pseudoarthrosis of long bones)
   HAROLD BOYD
   JEAN and ROBERT JUDET
   ROBERT D. RAY
   Discussion: 21 speakers

Symposium: L'enseignement de la chirurgie orthopédique et de la traumatologie et l'organisation des services dans les hôpitaux (Teaching and training in orthopaedic surgery and traumatology and the organization of hospital services)
Sir HARRY PLATT
ROBERT MERLE D'AUBIGNÉ
HAROLD A. SOFIELD
CARLO MARIO ZUCO
Discussion: 4 speakers

Free Papers: 31

Audio-Visual Programme: 34

Scientific Exhibits: 33

Officers of the Society

President: JEAN DELCHEF
Vice Presidents: JOSEPH TRUETA
F. E. GODOY MOREIRA
Secretary General: ANTOINE BAILLEUX
Treasurer: JOSEPH CORNET

►

Fig. 24. Some famous signatures on that souvenir menu ETIENNE SORREL, JOSEPH TRUETA, BRYAN MCFARLAND, PHILIP D. WILSON, PHILIP ERLACHER, ROBERT MERLE D'AUBIGNÉ, HARRY PLATT, R. I. HARRIS, JOSÉ VALLS and R. SOEUR

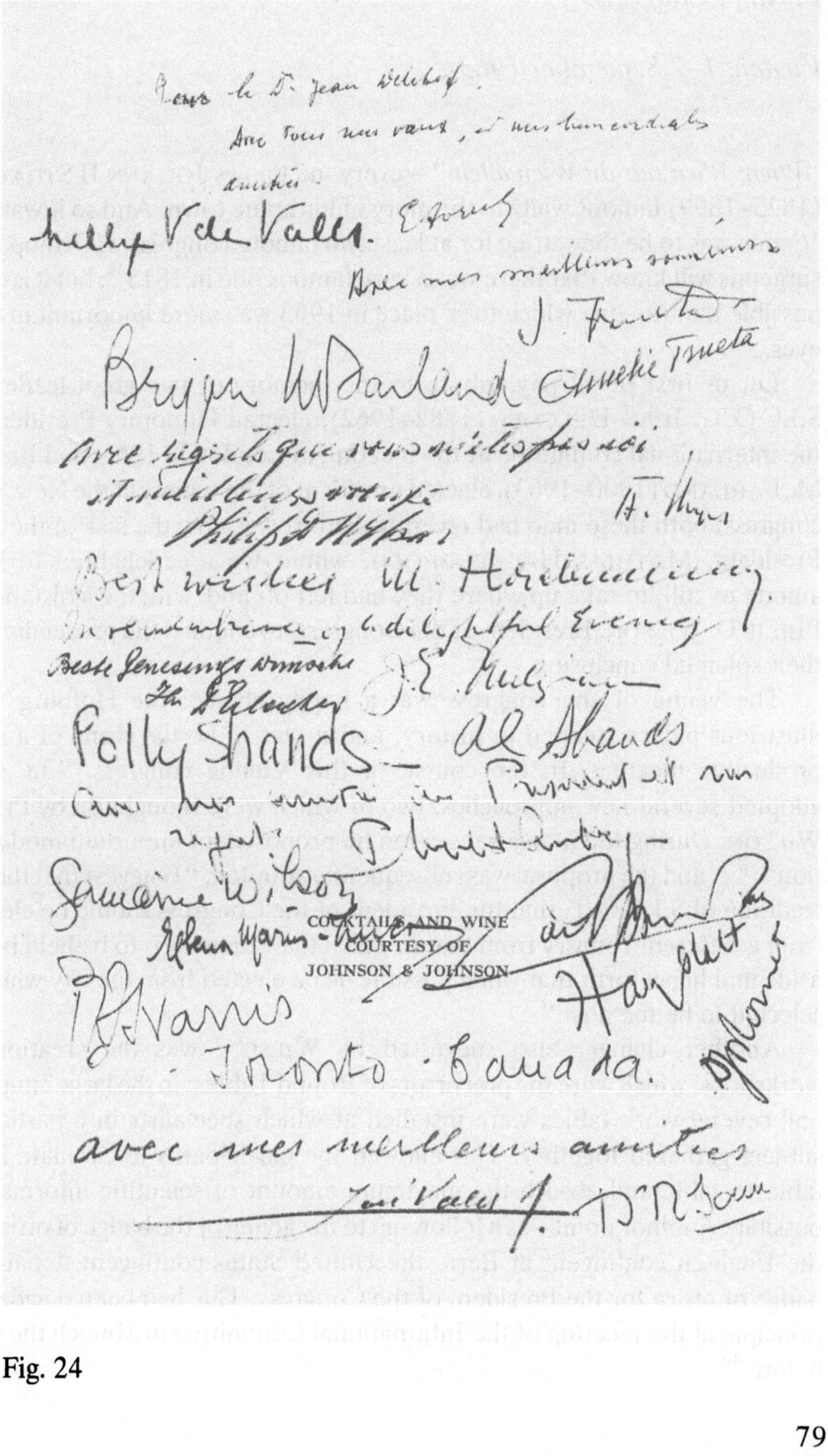
Avec mes meilleurs souvenirs
Best wishes
In remembrance of a delightful Evening
Polly Shands
Toronto · Canada.
COCKTAILS AND WINE
COURTESY OF
JOHNSON & JOHNSON
avec mes meilleurs amitiés

Fig. 24

F. Ninth Congress: "Joy"

Vienna, 1–7 September 1963[37]

"Wien, Wien nur du Wien allein" – everyone knows JOHANN II STRAUSS's (1825–1899) famous waltz to the glory of his home town. And so it was that Vienna was to be the setting for at least two famous congresses. Orthopaedic surgeons will know that there was a very famous one in 1815[38]; but it is quite possible that the one which took place in 1963 was more important in their eyes.

Let us first of all pay tribute to the memory of two great leaders of S.I.C.O.T., JEAN DELCHEF (1882–1962), elected Honorary President by the international committee at the meeting in London in 1961, and BRYAN MCFARLAND (1900–1963), elected president of the society at the New York congress; both these men had recently died. It was now the task of the Vice President, MATHIAS HACKENBROCH, whom we are delighted to have among us still, to take up where they had left off and, with the assistance of PHILIP D. WILSON, President of the Congress, to conduct the proceedings to their splendid conclusion.

The venue of the congress was a happy choice: the Hofburg[39], an illustrious palace steeped in history; and it was to be the scene of a most productive meeting. In the course of this Vienna congress, S.I.C.O.T. adopted several new approaches, two of which were thought up by PHILIP WILSON. During the inaugural session he proposed an important modification[37, p. 17] and the proposal was subsequently adopted: "I suggest that the old tradition of S.I.C.O.T. that the President of the Congress should be elected from a different country from that in which the Congress is to be held be set aside and henceforth that when possible he be elected from the city which is selected to be the host."

Another change, also suggested by WILSON, was the creation of workshops, which were the precursors of Round Tables; in the large congress hall several work tables were installed at which specialists in a particular subject gathered together. This allowed the participants to circulate from table to table and absorb the maximum amount of scientific information possible. A minor point – as a follow-up to the giving of the badge of office by the Englisch contingent at Bern, the United States contingent donated a badge of office for the President of the Congress. This had been decided in principle at the meeting of the International Committee in Munich the year before.[40]

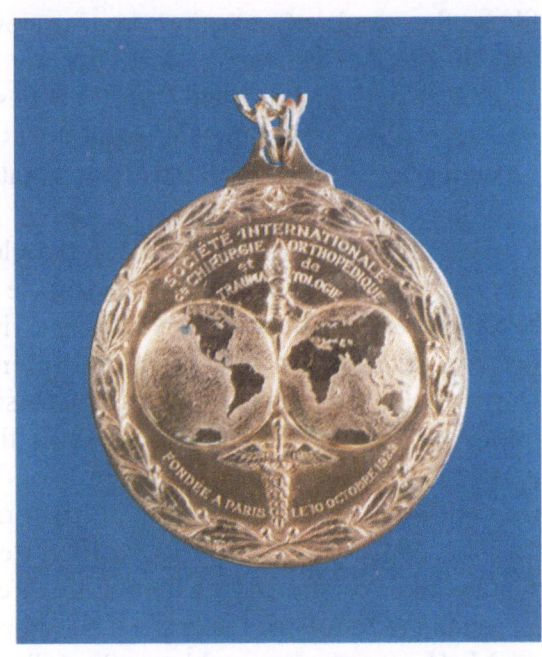

Fig. 25. The badge of office given by the U.S. section to the President of the S.I.C.O.T.'s meetings

It seems appropriate at this point to emphasise that the activities of S.I.C.O.T. are not limited to organizing a congress every three years. We have seen that there is also contact with other medico-surgical organizations and bodies. Since the foundation of the society the board of the international committee had met at least once a year. Increasingly, the boards has been holding a supplementary meeting, usually in the spring. In addition there are commissions which meet at the time of the congress to discuss audio-visual methods, classification, nomenclature, publications, scientific research (this particular commission has grown into an independant society, S.I.R.O.T., under the aegis of S.I.C.O.T.), the standardization of implants, and finally, statutes.

S.I.C.O.T. was growing in leaps and bounds: The total number of members had risen to 1100, and no less than 1000 people attended the congress. The scientific "harvest" was proportionate to this excellent attendance: 4 symposia, 61 audio-visual programmes, 19 stands of scientific exhibits and 68 free papers. Must we conclude from the increase in the number of free papers that the resolution passed at Barcelona had not been heeded? It is not clear, and the explanation is probably different; it was most likely the result of selection from an even greater number of papers submitted. The workshops arranged by Wilson brought together 103 specialists and experts. The "star" of these workshops was incontestably FRIEDRICH PAUWELS, that old magician, as one French surgeon dubbed him on seeing him at work. It was at Vienna that the surgery of osteotomy took a great leap forward.

The social events were just as one would expect from a city like Vienna. The reception at the town hall, given by the mayor, FRANS JONAS, who later became President of the state, left some vivid memories. A most colourful evening such as only Vienna can offer was spent at the Spanische Reitschule[41], and it was by no means necessary to be a horse enthusiast to be impressed by the spectacle. A walk in the outskirts of Vienna led the participants to the castle of SCHÖNBRUNN[42], and later to Grinzing to taste the delicious new wine *(Heuriger)*. A performance of "Tristan and Isolde" at the Staatsoper[43] is unlikely to be forgotten by the congress participants. Finally, the closing banquet held in the great congress hall of the Hofburg reflected the history of the city – it was imperial!

M. HACKENBROCH told me the following amusing anecdote: "I was sitting in the highest part of the theatre, known as 'paradise'; Sir HARRY had noticed this, and being seated in 'Olympus' himself along with the other leaders, had me descend to sit with him."

It was Sir HARRY PLATT again who, on meeting M. HACKENBROCH later in Paris (1966) signed sadly, "We're too old for all that now!" and HACKENBROCH retorted, "No, we just know too much about it..." (Personal communication from M. HACKENBROCH.)

Ninth Congress: Vienna, 1–7 September 1963

Officers of the Meeting

President:	PHILIP D. WILSON
Vice President:	PHILIP ERLACHER
Secretary:	KARL CHIARI
Assistent Secretary:	FRANZ ENDLER
Treasurer:	KARL-HERMANN SPITZY*

---

* Son of HANS SPITZY, a founder member.

Symposia

1. *The use of isotopes as bone markers* (L'usage des isotopes comme marqueurs osseux)
   Moderator: JOSEPH TRUETA

2. *Traitement chirurgical de l'arthrite rhumatoïde* (Surgical treatment of rheumatoid arthritis)
   Moderator: ROBERT MERLE D'AUBIGNÉ

3. *Traumatic lesions of the cervical spine* (Lésions traumatiques du rachis cervical)
   Moderator: OSCAR SCAGLIETTI

4. *The problem of embryonic malformations resulting from extraneous factors* (Le problème des malformations embyonnaires dues à des facteurs exogènes)
   Moderator: OSKAR HEPP

Free Papers: 68

Officers of the Society

Honorary President: JEAN DELCHEF †
President: BRYAN MCFARLAND †
Vice Presidents: MATHIAS HACKENBROCH
                   F. E. GODOY-MOREIRA
Secretary General: ANTOINE BAILLEUX
Treasurer: JOSEPH CORNET

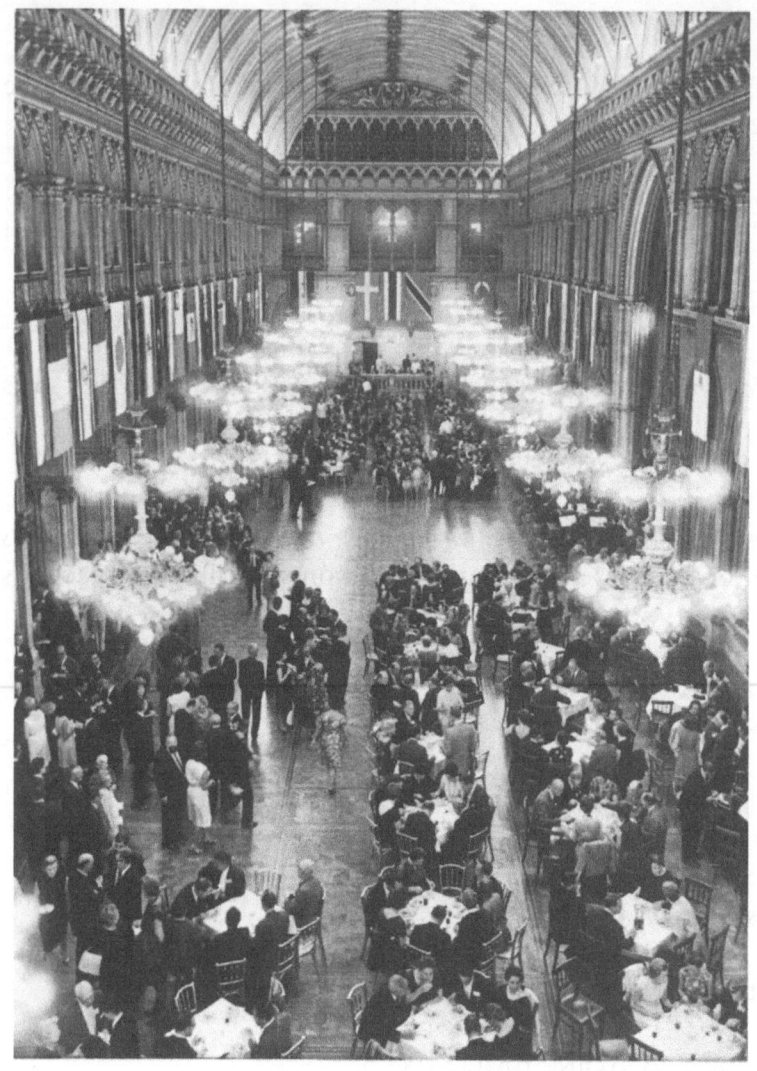

Fig. 26. The closing banquet at the Hofburg, venue of the ninth meeting

Paris, 4–9 September 1966[44]

In an international organization like S.I.C.O.T. it is always risky to pay a greater compliment to one country than to another, and it is not good form to spread the congratulations unevenly. Thank goodness – and pray God we may never descend to such things – we are not prone to inferiority complexes or petty nationalism; and so with a degree of diplomacy and reliance on scientific fraternity, due credit may be given for magnificent achievements. With these reservations, I think I am justified in saying that the tenth congress, held in Paris, was particularly successful. In a word, everything was raised to a higher level.

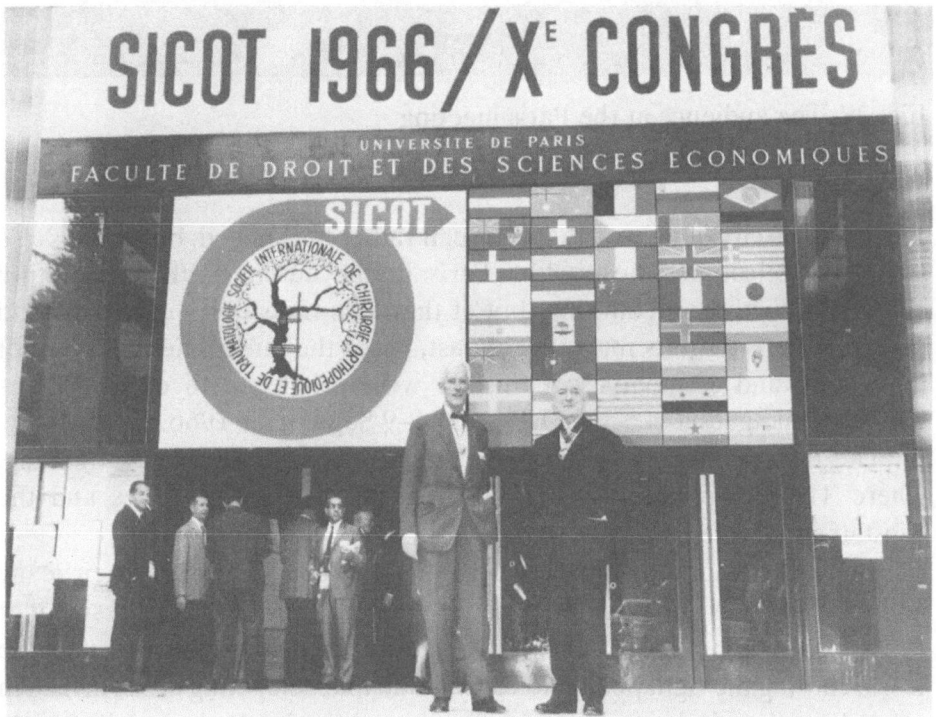

Fig. 27. The tenth meeting at Paris, when Themis hosted Aesculapius ROBERT MERLE D'AUBIGNÉ, President of the meeting and MATHIAS HACKENBROCH, President of the Society

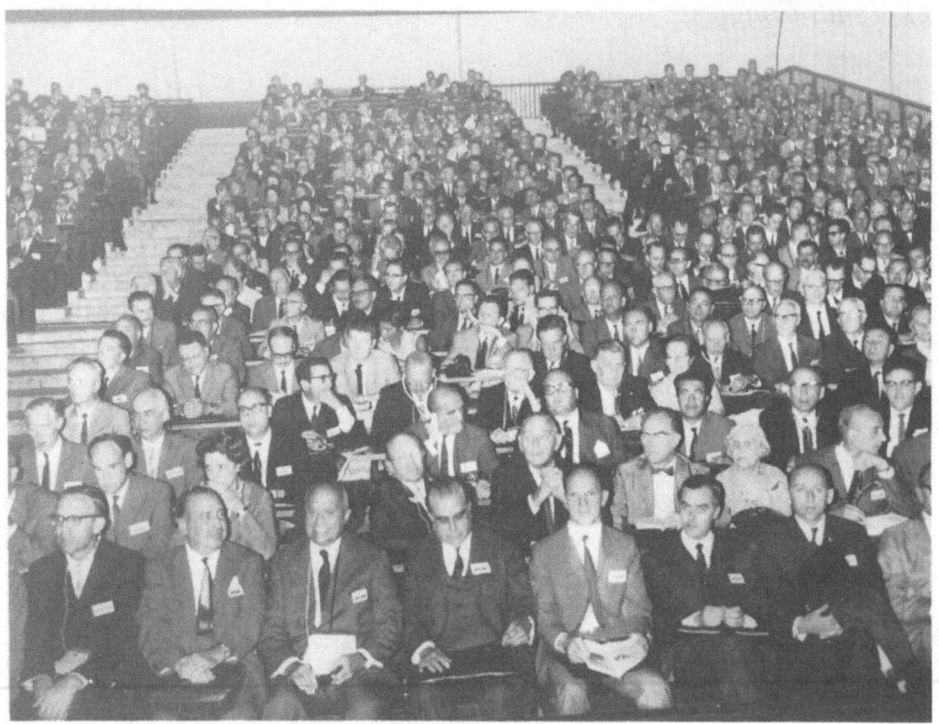

Fig. 28. The audience at the Paris meeting

Paris, the city of lights – that is true, if rather hackneyed; but Paris is also splendid, welcoming, hospitable. Paris in the autum, with its beautiful colours, seductive and alluring; but at the same time a hive of activity and research. Paris with its magnificent past, yet at the same time the cradle of innovation and creativity. All this we were privileged to experience as members and guests of S.I.C.O.T. from 4–9 September 1966.

The Faculty of Law in the rue d'Assas, a superb brand new building, where Themis graciously received Esculape, where the Scales and the Tipstaff stood side by side in harmony.

Our hosts made up an exceptional and energetic team, and their many and varied talents combined to produce a superb congress. The President of the Congress, ROBERT MERLE D'AUBIGNÉ, was an expert in planning the work, chosing the right people to carry it out, and delegating tasks; in fact, in controlling the whole procedure vigilantly and flawlessly. I am deliberately mentioning only the leader himself, because it is common knowledge that the captain of any team can be judged on the performance of his men; they work together as a unit, and as such have a right to our recognition and admiration.

In Paris between 4 and 7 September 1966 this particular team produced a remarkable display of work, progress, science and – entertainment.

The inaugural session was particularly fine, combining great delicacy of wit with a good deal of intellectual substance. The President of S.I.C.O.T., MATHIAS HACKENBROCH, paid tribute to our predecessors – our founders. The President of the Congress, ROBERT MERLE D'AUBIGNÉ, in a speech of considerable vision, expounded his thoughts on the orthopaedic surgery and the hospitals of the future, as well as his hopes for the way our special field would develop. Dr. BOULANGER, representing the French Ministry for Social Affairs, replied by thanking and congratulating the organizers of the congress, and afterwards gave a reception for the participants. The President of the Ordre des Médecins *(Society of Physicians),* Professor J. L. LORTAT-JACOB, honoured the ceremony with his presence.

After this the work began. Seven subjects were on the agenda and were examined in depth in the symposia or in general assembly without interest flagging for a moment. In giving an account of this congress, there are two items we should mention in particular: the extraordinary productivity of the Round Tables, and the closed circuit television system. The Round Tables, which had functioned admirably at the Vienna congress in 1963, reached their zenith during this Paris congress. There were so many factors which contributed to the deepening of the participants' knowledge: selection according to interest, the small number of obligatory attendances at these meetings, the fact that the speakers were authorities on their subject, to mention but a few. The closed circuit television system quietly and efficiently contributed to the comfort of all concerned. No one came to distract the attention of the auditorium when Mr. X was summoned, nor, on the other hand, when a communication of general interest had to be broadcast.

Thus it was possible for all to satisfy their thirst for knowledge; there were opportunities for individual meetings, which contributed to a very good atmosphere, and there was the scientific exhibition to visit.

We should also mention the first-class historical exhibition. The land which had nurtured PARÉ, ANDRY, DELPECH, LARREY, DUPUYTREN, MALGAIGNE, MAISONNEUVE and so many others was quite right to want to remember them in this way.

As may be expected, the social events were of the same high quality as the rest of the congress, with that touch of human warmth and hospitality so typically French. The first festivities took place at the Museum of French Monuments[45] where we were the guests of the organisers. On Tuesday 6 September there was a reception at the Cluny Museum[46], witness of centuries

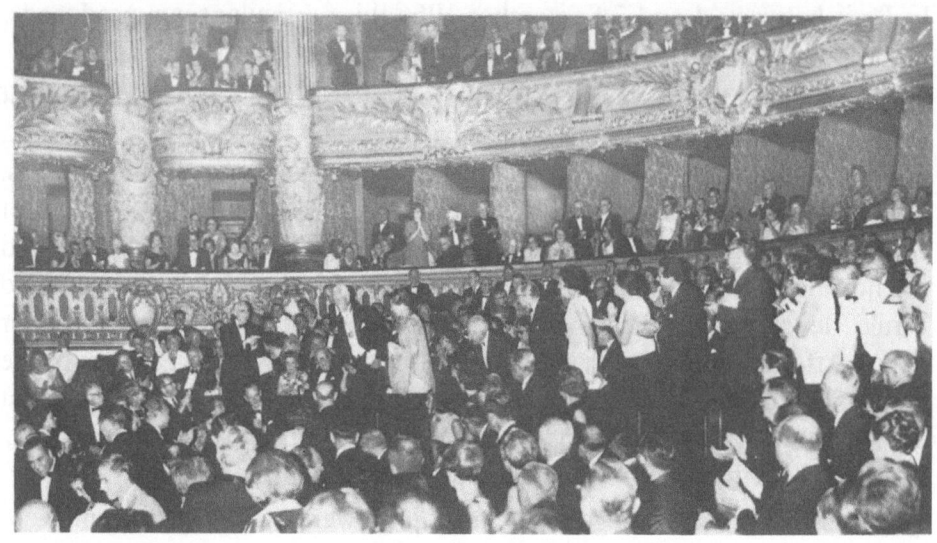

Fig. 29. A famous night at the Opera: the entry of the President of the meeting and Madame R. MERLE D'AUBIGNÉ

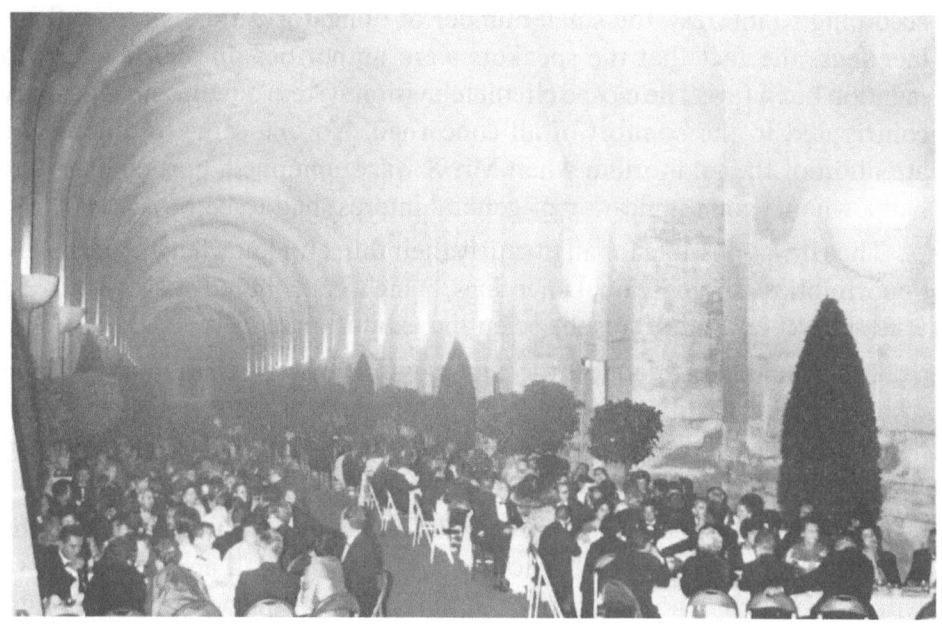

Fig. 30. The closing banquet at the Orangery of Versailles

of history. On Thursday 8 September the President and Madame ROBERT MERLE D'AUBIGNÉ were our hosts again, at the Opéra[47] for a private performance of "Carmen", the famous comic opera and masterpiece of its genre. The high point was indubitably the closing banquet on Friday 7 September, in the famous Orangery at Versailles.[48] Guest of honour was a government minister, Monsieur JEANNENEY. One statistic will give some idea of the enthusiastic response to this congress: there were 1400 places at table! And everyone returned home richer in scientific knowledge, with his spirit refreshed.

Note

JOSEPH CORNET, who had been running the finances of S.I.C.O.T. since the Barcelona congress, died at the beginning of 1966. ANTIONE BAILLEUX, JEAN DELCHEF's worthy and devoted successor as Secretary, was too ill to attend; and, making a definite mistake in his prognosis – most happily, since he is still with us – he conferred the post, with the approval of the International Committee and the general assembly, upon ROBERT DE MARNEFFE. Under the same conditions I took charge of the Treasury of S.I.C.O.T. and the post of Editorial Secretary was created and conferred upon JEAN DELCHEF, Jr.

Tenth Congress: Paris, 4–9 September 1966

Officers of the Meeting
President: ROBERT MERLE D'AUBIGNÉ
Vice President: PIERRE LANCE
Secretary: JACQUES RAMADIER
Treasurer: JACQUES DUPARC

*Subjects**

1. *Hanche traumatique de l'adulte* (Traumatic hip of the adult)
   Symposium No. 1: Biochmechanics of the femoral neck
   Moderator: CARL HIRSCH
   Symposium No. 2: Diagnosis of avascular necrosis

---

* As you may see, symposia had to be divided into Subjects with Symposia.

Moderator: HAROLD B. BOYD
Symposium No. 3: Revascularisation of the femoral head
Moderator: ROBERT JUDET
Symposium No. 4: Treatment of fractures of the cotyle
Moderator: E. A. NICOLL

2. *Hanche non traumatique de l'adulte* (Non-traumatic hip of the adult)
   Symposium No. 1: Early surgery in coxarthritis
   Moderator: ROBERT MERLE D'AAUBIGNÉ
   Symposium No. 2: Muscular divisions
   Moderator: CALOGERO CASUCCIO
   Symposium No. 3: Idiopathic necrosis of the femoral head
   Moderator: ROBERT MERLE D'AUBIGNÉ
   Symposium No. 4: Total prosthetic replacement for advanced cox-
   arthrosis
   Moderator: JOHN CHARNLEY

3. *Hanche non traumatique de l'enfant* (Non-traumatic hip of the child)
   Symposium No. 1: Normal development of the hip
   Symposium No. 2: Persistent displacement
   Symposium No. 3: Epiphysiolysis of the femoral head
   With conferences, free papers, etc.

4. *Greffes osseuses* (Bone grafts)
   Symposium No. 1: Biology of bone grafts
   Moderator: PIERRE LACROIX
   Symposium No. 2: Experimental study
   Moderators: PIERRE MAURER
               JEAN ZUCMAN
   Symposium No. 3: Hetero-grafts
   Moderator: R. MAATZ
   With conferences, free papers etc.

5. *Hand and upper limb*
   Symposium No. 1: Sutures and nerve grafts of the upper limb
   Moderator: Sir HERBERT SEDDON
   Symposium No. 2: Severe mutilations of the hand
   Moderator: RAOUL TUBIANA

Symposium No. 3: Intrinsic paralysis of the hand
Moderator: JOSEPH BOYES
Also conferences and free papers

6. *Spine*
Symposium: Final results in treatment of idiopathic scoliosis
Moderator: JOHN H. MOE
Also conferences and free papers

7. *Lower limb and miscellaneous*

Officers of the Society
President: MATHIAS HACKENBROCH
Vice Presidents: WALTER P. BLOUNT
                     ADAM GRUCA
Secretary General: ANTOINE BAILLEUX
Treasurer: JOSEPH CORNET †

Mexico City, 6–10 October 1969[49]

History shows some remarkable reversals. In 1521, HERNANDO CORTÈS (1485–1547) conquered Mexico; the epic is still famous.[50] Four and a half centuries later, it was the turn of the Mexicans to conquer the orthopaedic surgeons and traumatologists of the entire world. It was a conquest of a completely different nature, using the weapons of friendliness and smiles.

Mexico. It is hard to imagine a more complete change from European life: the climate, the altitude, the way of life, nature, archaeological treasures, ethnography – all this to be found not only in the town but also in the country. The Plaza Mayor or Zocalo, Chapultepec, Alameda[51], the Anthropological Museum – so many centres of cultural interest; but above all, the most striking sight for me was the Plaza de las Tres Culturas *(Plaza of the Three*

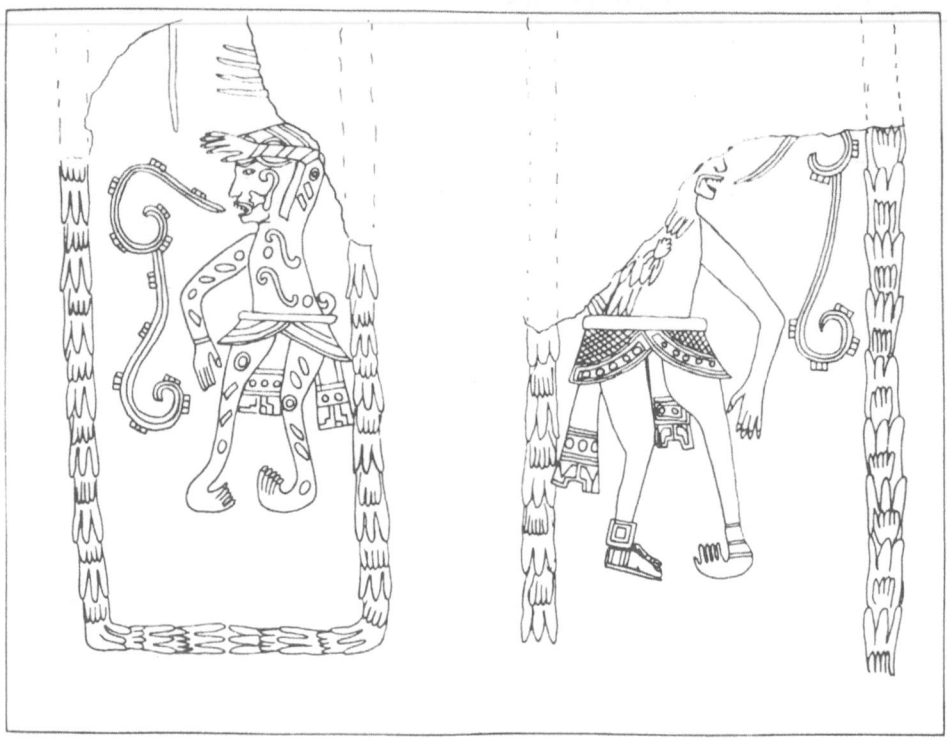

Fig. 31. Pre-cortesian Orthopaedics in Mexico (reproduction by kind permission of J.B.J.S.)

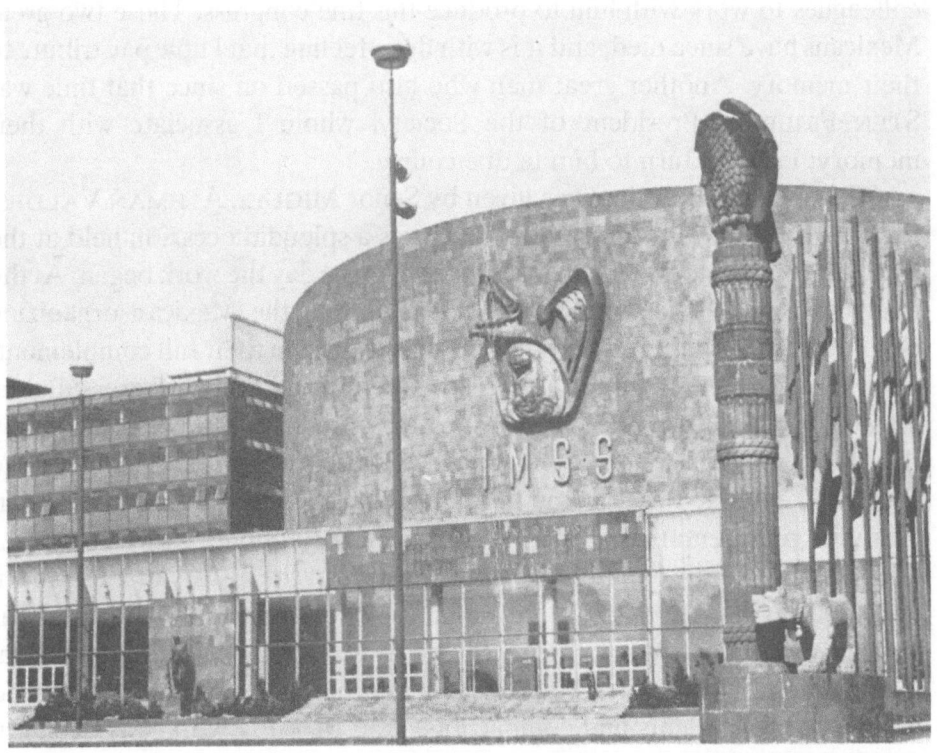

Fig. 32. The venue of the eleventh meeting in Mexico. Instituto Mexicano del Seguro Social (with kind permission of A. G. FORMENTI – Mexico)

Cultures) – Aztec, Spanish and Modern. It really is here that one finds the testimonies of the three civilisations which flowered in this part of the New World.

The Centro Medico Nacional, a superb edifice purpose-built for medical science meetings, was graciously put at the disposal of S.I.C.O.T. and the congress participants by the Rector of the University, JAVIER BARROS SIERRA. I was privileged to make the personal acquaintance of this aristocratic, and at the same time beneficent, gentleman, whose amenability and diplomacy had enabled him to remain in control of 80,000 students known for their vitality and their *machismo,* to use a local expression, for a great number of years – which was no mean feat. Personal contact with him was a most rewarding experience for me. In the same time I would like to mention Juan Farill, whom all his colleagues and compatriots called *"Maestro querido"* (dear Master) with veneration and respect. He was president of this congress. Kindness and dedication pesonified, always available and approachable, his wisdom was demonstrated in his choice of colleagues to work with him to produce this fine congress. These two great Mexicans have since died, and it is with deep feeling that I now pay tribute to their memory. Another great man who also passed on since that time was STEN FRIBERG, President of the Society, whom I associate with their memory; I shall return to him in due course.

The opening reception was given by Señor MIGUEL ALEMAN VALDES, President of the Council of Tourism. It was a splendid occasion held at the Hilton Hotel on Sunday 5 October. The following day the work began. At the inaugural session the officials of S.I.C.O.T. and the Mexican organizing committee were gathered together on the rostrum in their full complement, alongside representatives of the ministries concerned in the congress: Public Health, Social Security and Tourism. Musical interludes were provided by the choirs of the National University. STEN FRIBERG, President of the Congress, extended a welcome to all present, and invited Dr. SALVADOR ACEVES, representative of the President of the Republic, GUSTAVO DIAZ ORDAZ, to open the congress. In a brief outline of the history of medicine in his country, JUAN FARILL, President of the Congress, captivated his audience with what was for many their first acquaintance with the medical science of the Mayas. The Maestro querido charmed his guests, as he had done with his students and compatriots. And then the work was begun in earnest, centred on five main themes and 40 Round Tables, complemented by five stands of scientific exhibits. Two of these stands were particularly fine; one by the National Academy of Medicine, and the other by the Anthropological Museum. At a more general level, two master conferences* should be given particular mention. The first was given by JUAN FARILL on the theme "Orthopaedics and Psychology", at the beginning of the congress; and the second, presented by STEN FRIBERG at the end of the congress, was on "Students and Us" – his own particular area of competence. For STEN had been Rector of the University of Stockholm for 12 years, and was unique in its annals in his opposition to tradition. In the long rund this secured him the respect and veneration of his peers and students alike. He was a scientist of international repute, President of the Nobel Prize Committee for Medicine, consultant to the Ministry of Public Health in Sweden – the list is endless. These titles can only give some idea of the man. Personal contact with him was a most uplifting expeience for me; although he sometimes gave the impression of being a little cold, coming from the North, once you gained his conficence he was generosity and amiability personified.

---

* In actual fact this was an innovation which was to be adopted in subsequent congresses; it was the precursor of the S.I.C.O.T. Lecture.

The social events were far from disappointing; in particular we should mention the extraordinary Ballet Folclorico[52]; a son et lumière spectacle at the pyramids of Theotihuacan[53]; a Mexican soirée at Tepozotlan[54]; and a gala dinner on the premises of the old Faculty of Medicine. There was so much to see in the way of Mexican art and culture; and those who wished to extend their knowledge of archaeology and/or art had ample opportunity to do so – indeed they were spoilt for choice.

In a word, the congress was a resounding success.

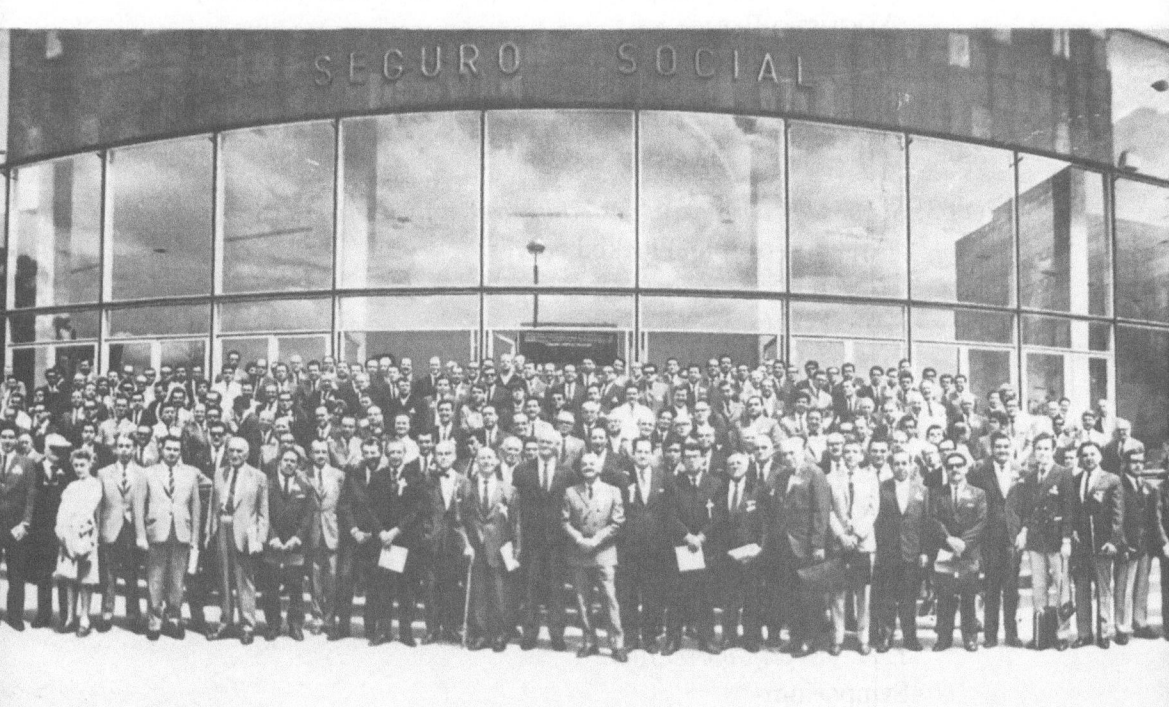

Fig. 33. The participants of the Mexico meeting in front of Instituto Mexicano del Seguro Social

Eleventh Congress: Mexico City, 6–10 October 1969

Officers of the Meeting
President: JUAN FARILL
Vice President: GUILLERMO DE VELASCO Y POLO
Secretary General: LEONARDO ZAMUDIO
Treasurer: MAX LUFT

Subject 1: *Survie au cours des accidents graves* (Survival and major injuries)
     GIORGIO MONTICELLI and PIETRO DI LEO
     ROBERT DE MARNEFFE and co-workers
     CARLOS E. DE ANQUIN
     Symposium

Subject 2: *Chirurgie reconstructive de la main et du membre supérieur*
     (Reconstructive surgery of the upper limb and the hand)
     AUGUSTO BONOLA
     JOSEPH H. BOYES
     Symposium
     Free Papers: 8

Subject 3: *Scoliose et correction des courbures spinales fixées* (Scoliosis and
     correction of spinal locked curves)
     Converences
     ADAM GRUCA
     PIERRE STAGNARA and co-workers
     WALTER P. BLOUNT
     Symposium
     Free Papers: 6

Subject 4: *La chirurgie de l'arthrose du genou* (Surgery of gonarthrosis)
     PAUL MAQUET
     MARK B. COVENTRY
     J. A. NOVA MONTEIRO
     Symposium
     Free Papers: 14

Subject 5: *Ostéosynthèse sous compression* (Compression internal fixation)
     Symposium
     Free Papers: 3

Subject 6: *Allongement et correction des inégalités de longueur des membres inférieurs* (Lengthening and correction of discrepancy in the length of the lower limbs)
Symposium
Free Papers: 6

Free Papers on General Subjects: Spine: 8, Hip: 20, Foot: 5, Fractures: 8, Miscellaneous: 17

Officers of the Society
President: Sten Friberg
Vice Presidents: Calogero Casuccio
  Karl Nissen
Secretary General: Robert de Marneffe
Treasurer: Edouard Vander Elst
Editorial Secretary: Jean Delchef, Jr.

I. Twelfth Congress: "Ardour"

Tel Aviv-Jerusalem, 9–13 October 1972[55]

We allow historians the privilege of passing judgement on the events of the past on two conditions: They must have irrefutable evidence, and a certain time lapse must have occurred.

Since I personally experienced both the events which led up to the choice of Tel Aviv for the 1972 Congress, and the Congress itself, I can bear witness myself. It is true that it was less than ten years ago that the International Committee met and the General Assembly in Mexico voted, and it could be argued that this time lapse is too short. But I feel that it would be an act of cowardice not to relate the troubles which arose on the occassion of this choice; and also, far worse, I would be depriving S.I.C.O.T. of a fine example of its work and its raison d'être.

97

Of course it was not the first time S.I.C.O.T. had encountered a problem of this nature; the account by Sir HARRY PLATT (p. 30) demonstrates this. The point is that in Mexico, Israel alone presented the International Committee with a structured programme worked out to its minute details. Italy was also in the running, but had not submitted a dossier as the rules required. The state of war in Israel constituted a serious objection to its being chosen as the venue for a congress, particularly three years before it was due to take place; and the arguments for and against were weighed up in all seriousness. In the end, M. HACKENBROCH, in a summing-up full of wisdom and serenity, helped us to decide: "How does the Europe of 1815 resemble that of 1969? My country is divided, and yet ... I did not oppose the creation of two German sections in the bosom of S.I.C.O.T. We should not waste our time on international political considerations." And so it was.

Italy, bearing witness to international friendship and solidarity above and beyond external events, in a gesture of great nobility offered to replace Israel in the event of the latter being unable to organize the 1972 Congress. Bravo for our Italian friends and members!

On the same subject, to go forward a little in time, I was deeply moved to see an Israeli member embracing an Arab friend and colleague at the Copenhagen congress in 1975. Many similar incidents demonstrate S.I.C.O.T.'s extraordinary capacity for forging links of friendship and uniting

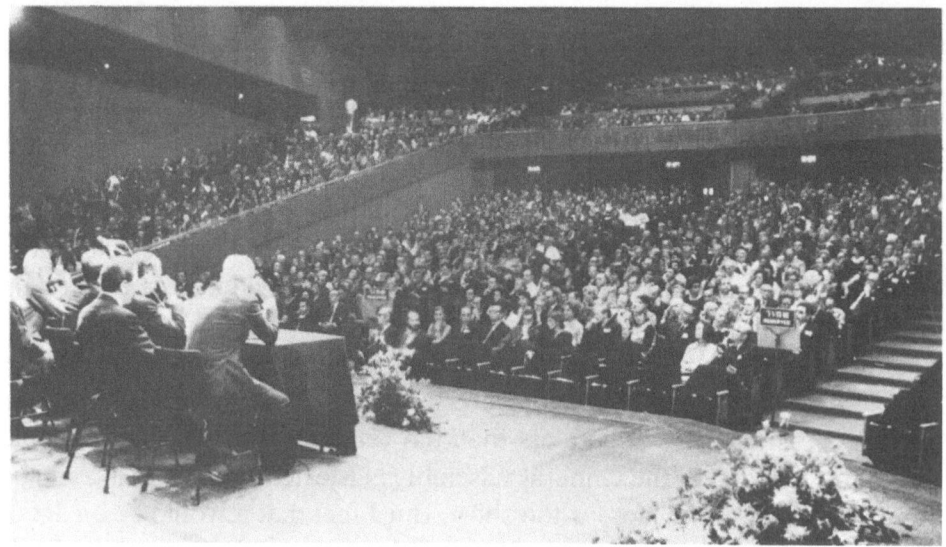

Fig. 34. The opening ceremony of the twelveth meeting at Tel Aviv in the Auditorium Mann

those who, outside her influence, are divided. Once more the "machine for fraternisation" was functioning well; the wishes formulated after the Amsterdam congress had been granted and the difficulties smoothed out; and I shall not be betraying any secrets if I add that the machine was to go on functioning well.*

Without recalling the difficulties mentioned above I would have been unable to recount these impressions imbued with human warmth and friedship, which is one of S.I.C.O.T.'s greatest assets. If I had not mentioned them, I would have been depriving S.I.C.O.T. of evidence of its vitality and of the ties that unite all its members. As it is, we have a pledge for the future for those who harbour any doubts.

Unfortunately – and this time I make no judgement – the events at the Munich Olympics[56] rather impaired the success and the efforts of our Israeli colleagues. There were many withdrawals and many absentees. Most fortunately nothing else went wrong and it was altogether an extremely fruitful congress.

It was very hot in Tel Aviv at this time, but not so as to inconvenience the participants, and the "Exhibition Gardens", a sort of open-air campus where the congress was held, were an ideal setting. Everyone adopted sub-tropical dress right from the informal introductory meeting, which took place during the day of Sunday 8 October on the congress site.

While the scientific work began the following morning, Monday 9 October, the inaugural session took place at 8.30 p.m. in the splendid FREDERIC MANN[57] Auditorium in the presence of representatives of the ministries of Education, Health and Tourism of the State of Israel. After welcoming these authorities, the President of the Congress, ERNST SPIRA, and the President of the Society, ROBERT MERLE D'AUBIGNÉ, spoke a few words to the participants. A most lovely concert was given, to the delight of the auditorium, which was estimated at at least 2000 persons. The Mayor of Tel Aviv/Yaffo gave a reception to round off the opening evening, which had equalled the climate in its warmth.

The following day the scientific work was begun, and in this connection we should recall two remarkable innovations brought about by the organizing committee. The first was the creation and conferring of fifteen fellowships for clinical or basic research to investigators all over the world. The prize consisted of a travel grant (regardless of place of residence) and

---

* A project in which S.I.C.O.T. is called upon to participate was a meeting of the Mediterranean Society for Orthopaedics and Traumatology with the participation of World Orthopaedic Concern in Cairo in 1979.

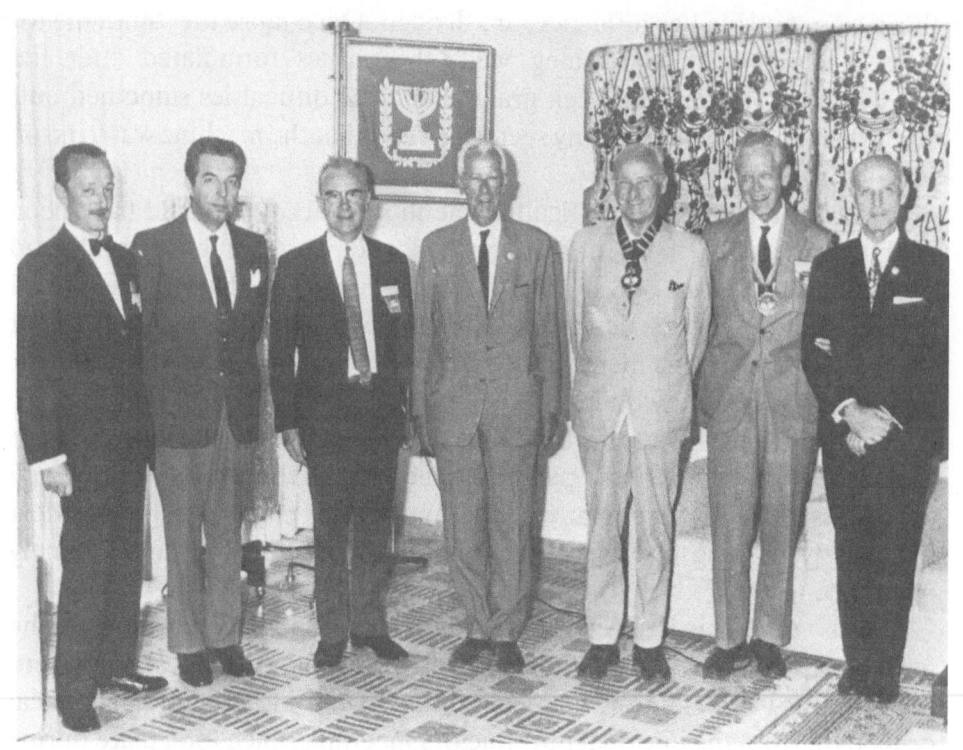

Fig. 35. The officers of S.I.C.O.T., guests of the President of Israel
ZALMAN SHAZAR (not here). From left to right:
JEAN DELCHEF Jr., Editorial Secretary
EDOUARD VANDER ELST, Treasurer
ROBERT DE MARNEFFE, Secretary General
ROBERT MERLE D'AUBIGNÉ, President S.I.C.O.T. 1969–1972
FLOYD H. JERGESEN, President S.I.C.O.T. 1972–1975
KNUD JANSEN, President S.I.C.O.T. thirteenth Congress
ERNST SPIRA, President S.I.C.O.T. twelfth Congress

accomodation expenses. Understandably this innovation was well received
and there were a great candidates. The second innovation was a series of
ideas to improve the presentation of the scientific programme and contribute
to the "classic" standard of the congresses. Here, too, the organizers met
with great success.

The next day the participants met at the amphitheatre of Caesarea, where
they were transported back twenty centuries in time. This was certainly of
great interest even to those who had little affinity for archaeology and
history.[58]

100

According to custom the closing banquet was the scene of farewells and adieus, and was at the same time the climax of the congress: a thousand guests assembled in the open air in the Exhibition Gardens – which for the past few days had been the scene of so much work – in an atmosphere of physical and spiritual well-being. The evening was enhanced by some very beautiful Israeli singing.

However, this banquet was not the end. On Friday 13 October all the participants were taken to Jerusalem to the "Binyanei Ha'ooma" (Palace of Congresses). There were two items on the programme: 1) The presentation of the diplomas to the fifteen award-winners, the first three of whom were to give a summary of their work on behalf of the group. 2) The second S.I.C.O.T. Lecture, a most illuminating conference with the world-famous archaeologist YIGAEL YADIN, who spoke very vividly and poetically on the epic of Massada.[59]

Finally the members of the board of S.I.C.O.T. were honoured in a way which reflected on all the members: They were given a private reception in the presidential palace by the Head of State, President ZALMAN SHAZAR.

My memories of this congress in the Holy Land are both delightful (as I have just shown) and moving, if not a little sad (as I shall now explain). In July 1976 I had written to ERNST SPIRA asking for some photographs as a souvenir of the congress which he and his colleagues had so splendidly and successfully arranged. Those who knew him well will not be surprised at his response: "…those pictures are smiling faces just similar to other congresses". The whole man is characterised in this reply – modest and humorous. Of course I pressed him further, and the reply came from his widow, MYRIAM SPIRA, whom we all remember for her humility and amiability. ERNST SPIRA having passed away in the meantime, "…on his desk we found the enclosed photographs, which we believe he assembled in response to your letter of July 8, 1976…"

Twelfth Congress: Tel Aviv, 9–12 October 1972

Officers of the Meeting
President: ERNST SPIRA
Vice President: MYER MAKIN
Secretary General: ITZAK FARINE
Treasurer: ALEXANDER KATZNELSON

Programme
1. *Fellowship Papers*
   BRIAN REEVES
   W. P. BOBECKO
   CARL L. NELSON
   HAJIME INOUE
   G. E. KEMPSON
   ERIC L. RADIN
   FRED LANGER and ALAN E. GROSS
   F. C. RILEY, JENIFER DOWSEY and D. BROWN
   SHOHEI MANABE and co-workers
   H. OONISHI
   CHARLES S. B. GALASKO
   R. SELIKTAR
   TZONY SIEGAL and ZVI H. MARCUS
   FRANZ BURNY and co-workers
   HIROMI AKATSU

2. *Symposia*
   Coxa plana
   The artificial hip joint and its biomechanics
   The rheumatoid hand
   Flexor tendon injuries
   Repair of injuries of peripheral nerves
   Osteoporosis of ageing bone
   Recent advances in malignant bone tumours
   Haemostatic deficiency surgery

3. *Free Papers:* 10 subjects

4. *Round Tables:* 5 subjects, each subdivided

5. *Innovations:* Preliminary reports on new concepts and ideas developed
   during 1972
   Clinical pathology conferences
   Diagnostic and technical tricks and pitfalls
   Brains trust
   History of orthopaedics

Note: It is impossible to give a full list of speakers.

102

Officers of the Society

President:	ROBERT MERLE D'AUBIGNÉ
Vice Presidents:	FLOYD H. JERGESEN
	KNUD JANSEN
Secretary General:	ROBERT DE MARNEFFE
Treasurer:	EDOUARD VANDER ELST
Editorial Secretary:	JEAN DELCHEF Jr.

*****

I have several times had reason to remark on the enthusiasm, confidence and energy of our founders. At Tel Aviv we were able to meet the two survivors of that team, PHILIP ERLACHER and PAUL LORTHIOIR, who were just as alert and agreeable as in 1929.

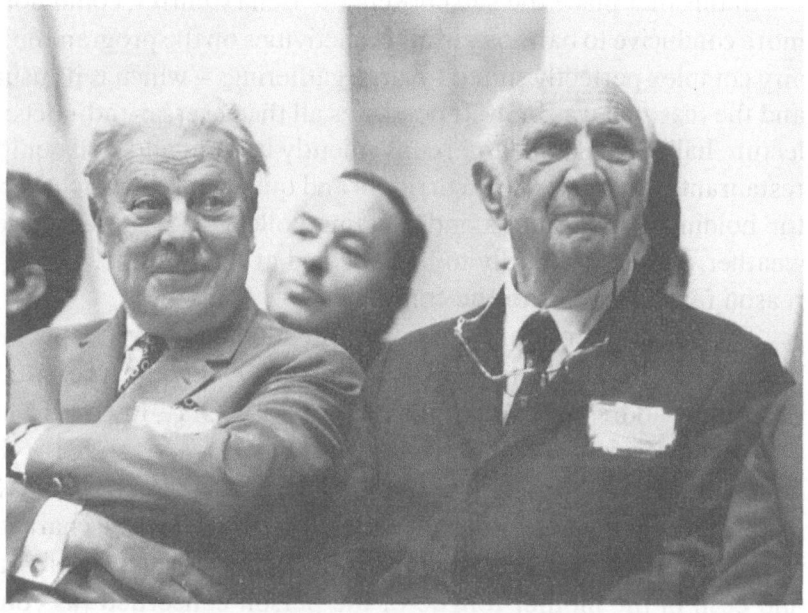

Fig. 36. PAUL LORTHIOIR and PHILIP ERLACHER. The two only surviving founder members, at Tel Aviv

103

J. Thirteenth Congress: "Friendship"

Copenhagen, 6–11 July 1975

There are some superstitious pessimists who consider the number 13 to be unlucky; while some superstitious optimists consider it to be a guarantee of success and good fortune. I must say that before the week of 6–11 July 1975 I was frankly indifferent to it; but during this week I ceased to be an unbeliever and became a superstitious optimist. In a word, the 13th congress was the cause of this change of heart.

S.I.C.O.T. Copenhagen 1975 was given the motto: "Friendship". Indeed, people call it "friendly Copenhagen"; and our Danish friends, led by KNUD JANSEN, certainly succeeded in giving the congress the air of relaxation and 'easy way of life' for which the Danes are renowned. As he said in his welcoming speech: "The spirit of our Congress shall also further the opportunities to renew old friendships and to create new ties. The Committee has made every effort to create an attractive frame and a worth-while week for you and your family".

In this first place the site chosen, the Bella Centret, could not have been more conducive to harmony in all the activities on the programme: It is a vast, airy complex perfectly suited to large gatherings – which is its usual function and the reason it was built. It possesses all the necessary adjuncts: functional lecture halls, small and large, conveniently laid out and well equipped; bars, restaurants, etc., and many corridors and quiet corners which were so useful for holding conversations and meeting colleagues. The exceptionally fine weather, which was hardly to be expected at this latitude, was an additional reason for the success of the congress.

The opening ceremony took place on Sunday 6 July at 4 p.m. in the great hall of the Bella Centret, with almost 1000 people present. After the welcoming addresses by the President of S.I.C.O.T., FLOYD H. JERGESEN, and the President of the Congress, KNUD JANSEN, JOHN FAIRBANK delighted the auditorium with the third S.I.C.O.T. Lecture, "A S.I.C.O.T. Profile". This was a colourful review of the historical characters of the society, each one being evoked by a particular trait or an amusing anecdote – and each in the mother tongue of the person concerned (as you may have guessed, JOHN FAIRBANK is a polyglot!). The whole lecture was shot through with British humour and perceptiveness. The final welcoming speech was

104

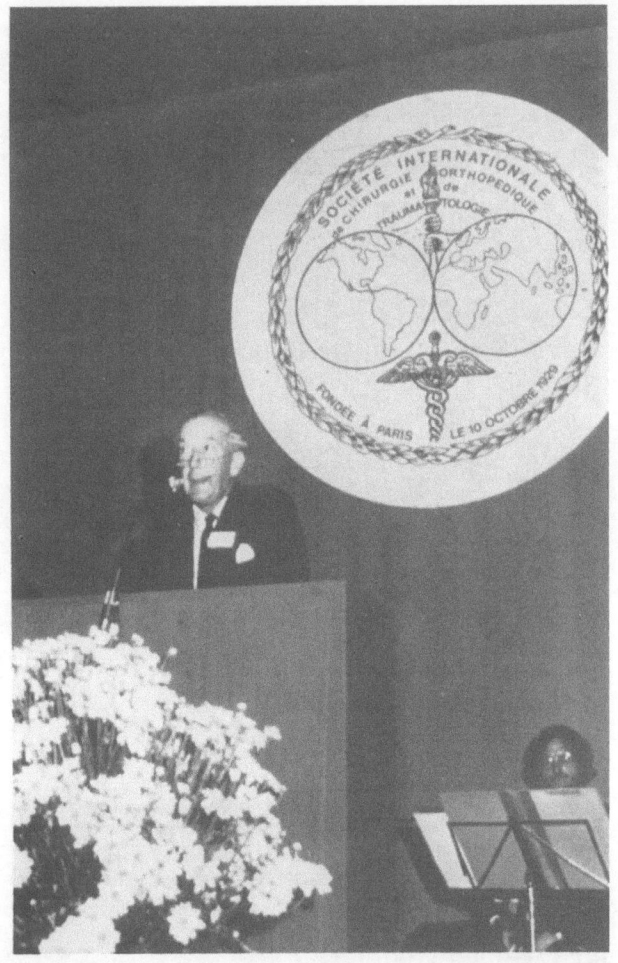

Fig. 37. Mr. JOHN FAIRBANK delivering the S.I.C.O.T. Lecture at the opening ceremony " A S.I.C.O.T. Profile"

given by Professor MORGENS ANDREASSEN, Rector of the University. Everything went according to plan, and the Tivoli Concert Hall Orchestra provided some pleasant musical interludes.

The same evening the participants met up in the oldest building of the University of Copenhagen, the Frue Plads[60]. It was not difficult to enter into the spirit of the traditions of the past, nor to remember that Copenhagen and its university had produced more than one scientiest for European medical science, whether anatomist, physiologist or practician: NIELS STEENSEN (1638–1786) who came to be known as NICOLAS STENON; the BERTELSEN

105

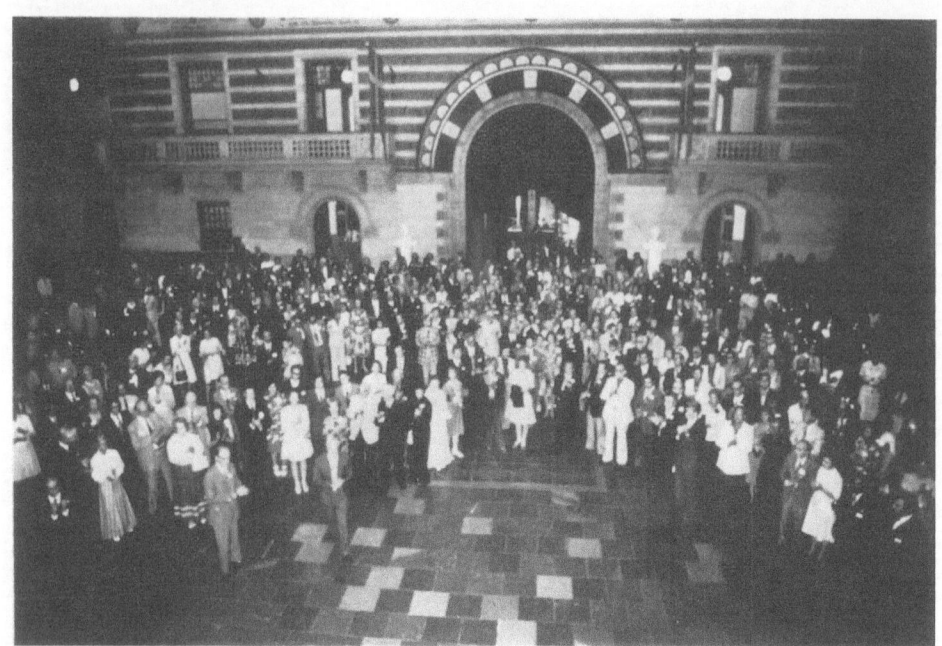

Fig. 38. Welcome get-together party, July 6, 1975 at the Ancient University of Copenhagen (Frueplads)

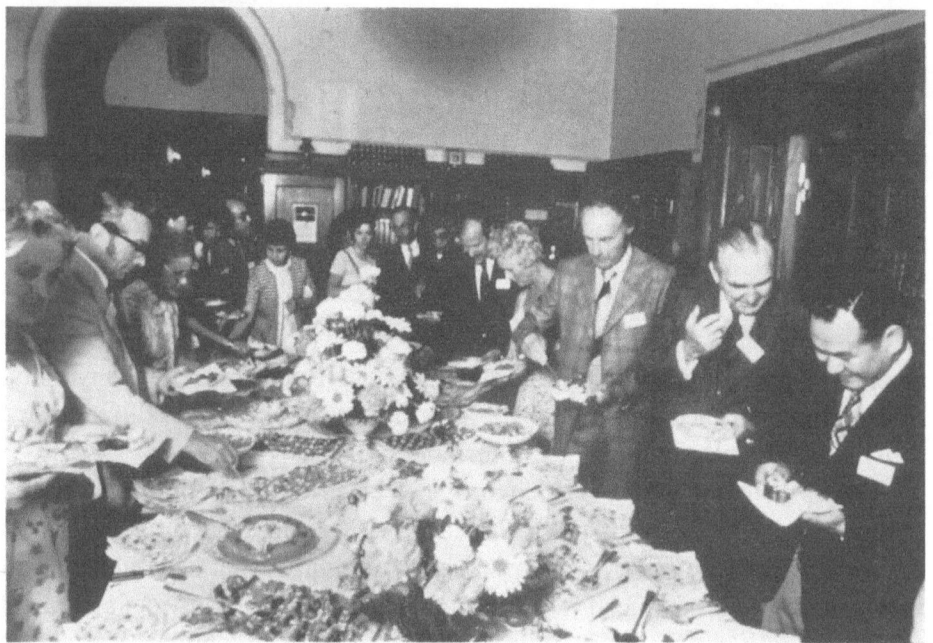

Fig. 39. The delicious Danish smörrebröds...

dynasty, the best known of whom was Tomas, later known as THOMAS BARTHOLIN (1616–1680), and finally and perhaps most famous of all, JACOB, later known as JACQUES (BÉNIGNE) WINSLOW (1669–1760). Incorrigible travellers – perhaps it was the Viking blood in them – they covered the whole of Europe, leaving wherever they went the traces of their hard work and many discoveries.

The next day everyone set to work; and this congress remained true to the best tradition in its grand scale, in the efficient organization, and in the large amount of scientific information disseminated. Twelve fellowship awards were rewarded with free travel access to the Congress and free accomodation, just as was done for the first time in Tel Aviv. The were 19 symposia, 20 instructional courses and almost 200 free papers, presenting those eager to learn with a choice that was at times difficult, and with constant variety. I should mention one particular innovation of this Copenhagen Congress: the Review Lectures. To this end, 16 authors particularly well versed in a topic of orthopaedic surgery were selected and invited by the organisers to "...present an outline of the progress through recent years within well defined fields of basic and clinical research". Along with the "Tricks and pitfalls", this was an addition to the list of innovations presented at Tel Aviv.

At this point we should note another progressive move by S.I.C.O.T. The 'proceedings' of the earlier congresses had reached such proportions that they had come in for some criticism. It was to alleviate this situation that the International Committee of Budapest in 1974 had decided in principle to found a review; and as we can see, those responsible did not waste any time in putting this idea into action. These Review Lectures were contained in a special issue of *Acta Orthopaedica Scandinavica,* and were the basis of what in the following months was to become *International Orthopaedics.*

As for the social events, there had been no let-up in the pace, and on the evening of Monday 7 July the participants divided up into three groups for receptions in three City Halls[61]: Copenhagen, Frederiksberg and Gentofte. Oh those delicious Danish cocktail snacks! Oh Tuesday 8 July, an enchanting evening was spent at Tivoli[62], famed throughout the world for its attractions for old and yound alike. Music lovers – and the rest – were delighted by a concert of classical music. The *piece de resistance* of this list of social events was without doubt the afternoon of Wednesday 9 July, when the servants of Science stopped work and were ready to relax. Two types of excursion had been arranged, in order to please everybody; and it was hard to make a choice, as there was so much to see: North Zealand, Frederiksberg Castle, Kronborg (Hamlet's) Castle and Fredensborg Palace[64], the Queen's summer residence; or Mid-Zealand, Roskilde Cathedral[66], Viking Ship Museum. In the evening everyone met up again at the Grundtvigskirchen[67] where the solemn beauty of a concert of religious music, enhanced by the excellent acoustics of the church, was appreciated by every-one.

The high point of the congress took place on Friday 11 July. After the closing ceremony, which is always a moving occasion with the passing on of offices, THORSKILD RAMSKOU revealed to us the secrets of the everyday life and the exploits of the legendary Vikings. In the evening, a supper attended by the dancers of the Danish Royal Ballet brought the congress to a close. No one will be surprised to hear that on the programme this event was entitled "Friendship Evening".

VOLTAIRE (1694–1778), the famous French writer, poet, moralist and pamphleteer, wrote: «*Les méchants n'ont que des complices; les voluptueux ont des compagnons de débauche. Les intéressés ont des associés. Les politiques assemblent des factieux. Le commun des oisifs a des liaisons. Les Princes ont des courtisans. Les hommes vertueux seuls ont des amis.*» (The wicked have accomplices; the voluptuous have fellow debauchees; mercenaries have associates. Politicians attract sedition-mongers; the idle have acquaintances; Princes have courtisans. It is only virtuous men who have friends.)

Many thanks to KNUD JANSEN and his colleagues on the Danish committee for showing that we are all virtuous.

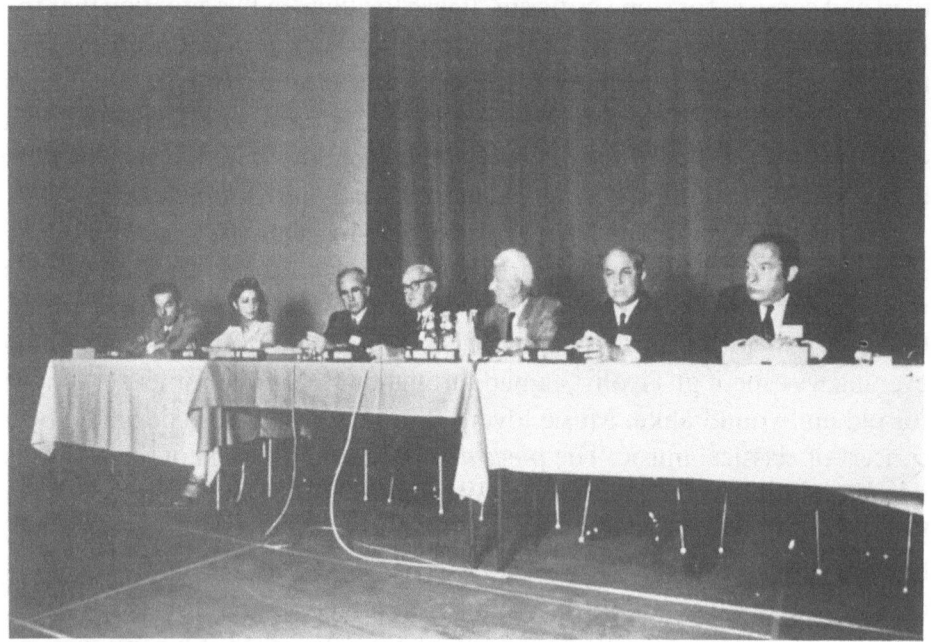

Fig. 40. S.I.C.O.T. Officers on duty...

108

Thirteenth Congress: Copenhagen, 6–11 July 1975

Officers of the Meeting

President: KNUD JANSEN
Vice President: EWIND THOMASEN
Secretary General: BENT EBSKOV
                               JØRGEN KJØBYE

Programme

1. *Review Lectures*
   Calcium metabolism: HECTOR F. DELUCA
   Tracer techniques in orthopaedics: GÖRAN BAUER
   Research in the pathology of osteoarthritis: CARL C. ARNOLDI and
   co-workers
   Genetics in orthopaedics: R. WYNNE-DAVIS
   Spinal dysraphism: JOHN LORBER and W. JOHN SHARRARD
   Management of the sequels of congenital hip dislocation: GEORGES
   MOREL
   Scoliosis: ROBERT WINTER
   Ankle lesions: CARL-AXEL CEDELL
   Hand reconstruction: RAOUL TUBIANA
   Biological reactions to physical forces in traffic accidents: PETER S.
   LONDON and C. VOIGT
   Biomechanics in sport injuries: VICTOR FRANKEL
   Spinal fractures: VERNON NICKEL
   Spondylolysis and spondylolisthesis: GIORGIO MONTICELLI
   Traumatic hip lesions: MARCUS STEWART
   Research and development within surgical amputee management:
   GEORGE MURDOCH

2. *Symposia*
   Osteosynthesis problems of stability: S. PERREN and MAURICE
   MUELLER
   Experimental studies of the electrical enhancement of bone healing: C. A.
   L. BASSETT

109

Spinal stenosis: JEAN CAUCHOIX
Cervical spine: T. MOROTOMI
Traumatology of the ankle: B. G. WEBER
Congenital dislocation of the hip:
Conservative management: GUNNAR WIBERG
Congenital dislocation of the hip:
Operative treatment: KARL CHIARI
Surgical implants: KNUD JANSEN
Orthopaedic training in developing countries: ANTHONY TRIAS
Management of orthopaedic infections: BERNHARD PAUS
Club foot: J. G. PETRIE
Rheumatoid arthritis: L. SOLOMON
Giant cell tumours: CARLOS OTOLENGHI
Bone healing: FLOYD H. JERGESEN
Arthroscopy: R. JACKSON
Bone metastases: LEON L. WILTSE
Arthrosis of the knee: GÖRAN BAUER, GIORGIO MONTICELLI
Scoliosis: ROBERT WINTER, J. HALL

3. *Instructional Courses*
Scoliosis, orthopaedic sepsis and many other subjects were expounded
and discussed, and there were numerous free papers and Round Tables.

Officers of the Society

President: FLOYD H. JERGESEN
Vice Presidents: CARLOS OTOLENGHI
                     WILLY TAILLARD
Secretary General: ROBERT DE MARNEFFE
Treasurer: EDOUARD VANDER ELST
Editorial Secretary: JEAN DELCHEF, Jr.

Notes

1. The Place de la Concorde is certainly one of the most beautiful plazas in the world, and was opened on 20 June 1763 next to the Tuileries Gardens. At that time it was called Place Louis XV. In the centre, King Louis XV (1710–1774) sits on horseback, surrounded by four statues: Peace, Prudence, Might and Justice. A scurrilous little ditty immediately went into circulation:

> *Ah, les belles statues, le beau piedestal*
> *les vertus sont à pied, le vice est à cheval.*

This was a direct allusion to the dissolute life led by the king. A free translation runs like this:

> Oh, nice statues, nice king
> virtues are standing vice is horseriding.

During the revolution, it was the scene of some bloody events, and a scaffold was permanently erected there, on which Louis XVI, Marie Antoinette, Louis Philippe Egalité and Madame du Barry were beheaded, among others. By a law of 26. 10. 1795 it was given its present name: Place de la Concorde.

The Hôtel Crillon was for a long time the Parisian residence of an illustrious family of captains and men of war in the service of the French crown. Louis de Crillon (1543–1615), whom King Henry IV (1553–1610) had proclaimed the best captain in the world, received the following brief and flattering note from his king: "Hang yourself, good Crillon, we have won the battle of Arques, and you were not there". This illustrates to posterity the regret felt by great valiant hearts at being absent at the time of a victory – and this is precisely what happened to Jean Delchef, as we have seen.

2. This list is in accordance with the S.I.C.O.T. archives and consists of twenty-one names. On the photograph Jean Delchef does not appear, as he was too ill; nor does Louis Rocher, for reasons unknown. *N.B.* Neither Fairbank (4) nor Meyerding (5) give the correct list.

3. The meeting at the Hôtel Crillon was in fact the result of long negotiations in which Anglo-Saxon surgeons from both sides of the Atlantic played an important part. The S.I.C.O.T. archives have carefully preserved the many letters and documents exchanged on this subject, some of which may be seen at the commemorative exhibition at this Kyoto congress. This meeting was the subject of two accounts, one by Sir Thomas Fairbank (undated) and the other by Henry W. Meyerding, dated 20 October 1929 in Berlin. These documents complement each other, which is why we felt it would be interesting to reproduce them here.

111

4. Account written by Sir THOMAS FAIRBANK (undated)
Meeting in Paris to form an International Society of Orthopaedic Surgery
October 10th and 11th 1929
Present
Dr. ALBEE, New York (in the chair)
Dr. PUTTI, Bologna
Dr. JANSEN, Leiden (unofficial secretary and interpreter)
Dr. ERLACHER, Austria
Dr. SPITZY, Vienna
Dr. JEAN JIANO, Bucharest
Dr. R. SAN RICART, Barcelona
Dr. J. ZAHADNICKY*, Prague
Dr. HAGLUND, Stockholm
Dr. MACHARD, Switzerland
Dr. GALEAZZI, Milan
Dr. SORREL, Paris'
Dr. MAFFEI, Brussels
Dr. LANGE, Munich**
Dr. BIESALSKI, Berlin**
Dr. WALDENSTRÖM, Stockholm
Dr. OMBREDANNE, Paris
Dr. MEYERDING, Rochester, Minnesota
Dr. BAER, Baltimore
Dr. NOVÉ-JOSSERAND, Lyon**
Mr. FAIRBANK
Dr. LORTHIOIR, Brussels

The British Memorandum was handed to Dr. ALBEE and read out, first in English and then in French. It was a bombshell. There was not a single supporter. I explained that the memo must not be taken as a blunt declaration that the British Orthopaedic surgeons would have nothing to do with the thing whatever, supposing it were decided by the meeting to form a new Society, but that it expressed a very strong feeling against the advisability of forming a new Association. I gave additional reasons for our opinion, particularly emphasizing the effect on the national meetings. The new Association must affect adversely the younger men who would not be eligible for election to it. I told them of the enormous number of medical meetings already open to British orthopaedists, and of the fact that the International Society of Surgeons was not well attended by the British surgeons, and I thought the same thing would happen with the new society, if formed. Also real discussion was impossible in a large society consisting of many members from many nations, and that much time was wasted.

---

   * Should read "Zahradnicek"

** LANGE and BIESALSKI were not present at the Hôtel Crillon on October 10, as they do not appear on the official photograph; unless they were present the day after, but I was unable to confirm this. The same applies to NOVÉ-JOSSERAND, of Lyons, who is not recorded as a founder member. On the other hand, LOUIS ROCHER, of Bordeaux, who does not appear on the photograph, is nevertheless recorded as a founder member. (See note 2.) VdE

Dr. PUTTI took a leading part in the discussion which followed: there was never any doubt about the result. All these men had come from all over the continent with the intention of forming a new Society, and our standing out would have made no difference, except a little soreness. I had to admit that I thought most, if not all, of the British Orthopaedic surgeons nominated for the International Society would accept election, but I was afraid their attendance would be poor. If the meetings were held at sufficiently long intervals, certainly not less than once every three years, this would go a long way to meet our main objections.

It was decided to form an International Society of Orthopaedic Surgery ("of Bone and Joint Surgery" was rejected).

A vote for holding meetings every three years against every five years resulted in favour of three years, but it was by no means an unanimous decision. It was decided to frame the By-Laws on those of the International Society for Surgery, and in spite of the late hour and protests led by Putti and myself, they proceeded to discuss each rule in turn. Small groups were chatting all round the room, taking refreshments during much of this. (The meeting started just after *10.45* and finished at 1 a.m.) The Executive is to consist of the President, Treasurer and Secretary, and one member of each country. Nomination for election to be made (forthwith) by a small nomination Committee of 3 in each country. For the British Elmslie (as President of the British Orthopaedic Association), PLATT and myself were chosen, and a complete list for all the nations was made out (and later lost). One of the three is to be the delegate on the Executive Committee.

It was finally decided to leave the discussion of further points to a small Sub-committee consisting of Dr. ALBEE, PUTTI, OMBREDANNE, SPITZY, JANSEN and myself.

We met at 9 a.m. next morning and decided the main points. These decisions were submitted to another meeting of many (not all) of the delegates at 6 p.m., and further points were decided. *These decisions were:* – that Sir ROBERT JONES be invited to become President of the International Society and also President of the first Congress to be held in Paris next year. (The latter was my suggestion, as Sir ROBERT is the only man who can be considered as international.)

Vice Presidents: Dr. PUTTI, Dr. GOCHT (Berlin)

Treasurer: Dr. MAFFEI

Secretary: Dr. DELCHEF   of Brussels

The office and secretarial organization of the International Society of Surgery are available for the new Society.

The first meeting to be in Paris on June 5th and 6th 1930 (just before the Whitsun holidays) provided Sir ROBERT can manage this. (This was decided only after long discussion, and in spite of any protests from me). Membership to be limited to 100.

To begin with the following nominations are asked for, each nation being invited to send in more than the allotted number (i.e. half as many again) arranged in order of merit.

Subjects for discussion at the first Congress were suggested:

1. Congenital dislocation of the hip:
   a) Treatment after age of election
   b) Results of treatment at all ages.
2. Injuries in the region of the wrist joint.

Finally it was left to the President and the two Vice-Presidents to decide.

Membership of the Various Nations

England	10
America	10
Italy	10
Austria	3
Germany	10
Belgium	3
France	10
Switzerland	3
Sweden etc. and Denmark	5
Roumania	3
Spain	3
Czechoslovakia	3
Holland	3
Russia	3
	79

Nomination Sub-Committee for Each Nation

Germany	Lange	Biesalski	Gocht
Austria	Erlacher	Spitzy	Wittel
America	Albee	Meyerding	Baer
England	Elmslie	Fairbank	Platt
Belgium	Delchef	Lorthioir	Maffei
Spain	San Ricart	Bastos	Ribo
France	Ombredanne	Sorrel	Nové-Josserand
Holland	Jansen	Franche	Van Assen
Italy	Putti	Galeazzi	Della Vedova
Roumania	Jean Jiano	Belacasco	Juvara
Sweden	Haglund	Waldenström	Bentrova
Switzerland	Meord	Scherb	Machard
Czechoslovakia	Chlumsky	Springer	Zahzadnicky

5. Account written by Dr. MEYERDING
Hotel Adlon, Berlin W.
Unter den Linden 1
Am Pariser Platz
Oct. 20, 1929

Dear Doctor MAFFEI,
The included notes were made by me at the International Society of Orthopaedic Surgery, and
I am sending them to you as I promised in Paris. The notes are of course incomplete due to my
inability to follow the several discussions going on at once in different languages.

114

The included notes were made by me at the Hotel Crillon, Paris Oct. 10, 1929.
The following men gathered at the Hotel Crillon by invitation to discuss the organization of an
International Society of surgeons at 10.00 p.m. on Oct. 10, 1929:

1 ROCHER, Bordeaux
2 SORREL, Paris
3 MAFFÉI, Brussels
4 PUTTI, Bologna
5 FAIRBANK, London
6 ALBEE, New York, U.S.
7 BAER, Baltimore, U.S.
8 MEYERDING, Rochester,
   Minnesota, U.S.
9 GALEAZZI, Milan
10 WALDENSTRÖM, Stockholm

11 JANSEN, Leiden
12 OMBRÉDANNE, Paris
13 FRANZ*, Bucarest
14 ZAHRADNICECK, Czechoslovakia
15 RICART, Barcelona
16 SPITZY, Vienna
17 ERLACHER, Graz
18 HAGLUND, Stockholm
19 LORTHIOIR**, Brussels
20 MACHARD**, Geneva

These men, after waiting for Dr. ALBEE about 45 minutes, elected Dr. MURK JANSEN
temporary chairman and Dr. BAER was given the floor. He suggested membership should
include general surgeons who had contributed to the advance of bone and joint surgery as well
as orthopaedists and surgeons of children, and after general discussion, it appeared to be
acceptable to all. Dr. ALBEE came in and was ask(ed) to take the chair, and Dr. JANSEN to act
as secretary. As all present could not speak or understand a common language, French and
English were interpreted by Dr. JANSEN and later Dr. PUTTI. Dr. ALBEE then said the English
orthopaedists had sent a letter by Mr. FAIRBANK, which should be read and discussed.
Mr. FAIRBANK: "The letter is only an expression of opinion and (though?) the English were
not in favour of an international organization they would join if one was formed.
Dr. PUTTI then answered the attitude of the English and said "There is no objection to the
formation of this society, we are here and now is the time to organize". (All present seemed to
agree.) PUTTI then advised starting with a small membership consisting of those present as
charter members and gradually enlarging the organization, the older men to lead the younger
in serious work (applaud).
FAIRBANK suggested meetings every three years (agreed). The discussion then continued
about the English attitude.
PUTTI stated he didn't think they were against it, except for the "splendid isolation of
England".
ALBEE: everyone in favour but the English. He suggested that starting with the members
present the society be increased to 100. 10 from large countries, to be nominated after
election. He suggested one decision on a name, draw up a constitution and form the
organization, then turn of minor details to a Committee (agreed).
SPITZY says the German orthopaedic society agrees to the organization of the International.
He acts as representative. The membership should not be nominated by the national surgical
or orthopaedic societies. A Committee of each country to nominate but election should be
made by the men present as charter members.

---

* Obviously a mistake, as it is known that Jiano is concerned.
** The last two names, omitted by Meyerding, have been added by Maffei in pencil. The list is
   correct, DELCHEF, as already mentioned, being absent due to illness. (VdE)

HAGLUND: Small countries will have difficulties in electing men.

SPITZY: No difficulties: the present organization elects, the Committee nominates. Good men are always outside national organizations for various reasons, and we avoid politics by electing new men nominated by a Committee made up now from the present membership etc. ...

PUTTI: We have accomplished our purpose, let organize and adapt etc. ...

ALBEE and JANSEN then made and interpreted in English and French with PUTTI and SPITZY from the International Surgical Society constitution which SPITZY had brought and the following were voted and passed after considerable discussion:

NAME: International Society of Orthopaedic Surgery. Object is to further orthopaedic surgery.

Membership is restricted; the present members begin the Society as charter members. Each country appoints three members; one to be delegate elected by the three. These delegates constitute the International Committee and they determine every three years before the meeting the number of members for each country.

The society is ruled by a permanent international Committee consisting of the President, Vice-Presidents and delegates. This committee elects its president from among the members.

A meeting to be held every three years.

German, French, English, Italian and Spanish languages to be used. *All officers are honorary* Triannual dues $ 10.00 or equivalent

A committee is appointed to perfect by-laws etc. ...: SPITZY, PUTTI, JANSEN, FAIRBANK, OMBREDANNE.

Dr. MEYERDING: the dues be paid in and Dr. MACHARD act as temporary Treasurer. Photograph which had been taken to be paid for from Treasury and copy sent to each member. Meeting adjourned.

Drs. JANSEN, SPITZY and MEYERDING met later 2.00 a.m. and went over constitution translating German to English from International Surgical.

6. Histoire de la Chirurgie Orthopédique et de la Traumatologie. E. VANDER ELST in: Histoire Générale de la Médecine, Vol. V. Editions ALBIN MICHEL, ROBERT LAFFONT et TCHOU, Paris. In press.

7. Vol. 1 "Procès-verbaux, Rapports et Discussions du Premier Congrès de la Société Internationale de Chirurgie Orthopédique". (Proceedings of the First Congress of the International Society of Orthopaedic Surgery; Vol. 1.) Brussels: R. Fischlin, 1931.
The Amphithéâtre Vulpian is situated in the old Faculty of Medicine, 12 rue de l'Ecole de Médecine, Paris.

8. S.I.C.O.T. archives, note by Sir HARRY PLATT.

9. Vol. 2 "Procès-Verbaux, rapports et discussions et communications particulières" du Deuxième Congrès International de Chirurgie Orthopédique". (Proceedings of the Second Congress of S.I.C.O.T.; Vol. 2.) Brussels: Lielens, 1933.

10. WILLIAM JOHN LITTLE (1810–1894), a London neurologist, who himself suffered from club foot, allowed himself to be operated on by GEORG FRIEDRICH STROMEYER (1804–1876) and, delighted by the results, in 1837 founded what was to become the Royal National Orthopaedic Hospital.

116

11. Details of the collections of the Royal College of Surgeons of England are to be found in the *Journal of Bone and Joint Surgery,* Vol. 36 B, No. 2, May 1954, pp. 323–331; and Vol. 36 B, No. 3, August 1954, pp. 490–495.

Sir HARRY PLATT also gives some interesting details in "Royal College of Surgeons of England" Hunterian Festival, 1955, pp. 89–93 in "Selected Papers". Edinburgh and London: E. & S. Livingstone, Ltd., 1963.

The Hunterian Museum – the collection of JOHN HUNTER (1728–1793) – is housed in the College. The College Library contains some 150,000 volumes.

12. The organization of medicine and surgery began to be codified in London at the beginning of the sixteenth century. KING HENRY VIII (1491–1547) in 1522 and 1523 promulgated the charter of the "College or Commonalty of the Faculty of Physick of London" which in 1851, under Queen VICTORIA (1819–1901) became the Royal College of Physicians. The surgeons had a difference of opinion with the barbers, from whom they officially separated around 1790. In 1800, King GEORGE III (1738–1830) granted them the charter of the Royal College of Surgeons of London, which in 1843 became the Royal College of Surgeons of England.

13. Vol. 3 Procès-verbaux, rapports, discussions et communications particulières Troisième Congrès International de Chirurgie Orthopédique. (Proceedings of the Third International Congress of S.I.C.O.T.) Brussels: Lielens, 1937.

14. Journal of Bone and Joint Surgery, Vol. 32 B, No. 4, 1950, pp. 570–586. "Orthopaedics in Continental Europe", Sir HARRY PLATT. Also in "In memoria di Vittorio Putti". Francesco Delitala, *Chirurgia degli Organi di Movimento,* Vol. 24, 1941. The Putti Foundation comprises 2457 old books and 1373 modern ones, not to mention innumerable periodicals, offprints, letters, etc. There are also 379 autographs of celebrated physicians, approximately 200 medals, ancient and modern surgical instruments, engravings, theses, photographs, etc.

15. Société Internationale de Chirurgie Orthopédique et de Traumatologie. Report by Sir HARRY PLATT. *Journal of Bone and Joint Surgery,* Vol. 30 B, No. 3, August 1948, pp. 408–409.

16. Sir HARRY PLATT: "A Running Commentary by Peripatetic Correspondents". *The Lancet,* May 11, 1948.

17. Réunion à Bruxelles, 2–5 octobre 1946, Procès Verbaux, necrologie, rapport, discussion, communications particulières. (Proceedings of the Brussels Meeting, 2–5 October 1946.) Brussels: Lielens, 1950.

18. Vol. 4 Procès Verbaux, rapports, discussions et communications particulières. (Proceedings, Vol. 4.) Brussels: Lielens, 1950.

19. Journal of Bone and Joint Surgery, Vol. 30 B, No. 4, Nov. 1948, pp. 725–730. I did not want to add anything to this account, but I feel that I should point out that the volume of "Proceedings" (note 18) contains many other details, in particular in the report by the Secretary General, JEAN DELCHEF; in the welcoming address by the Rector of the University,

117

Dr. G. C. Herringa; and in the address by the President of the Congress, Henry W. Meyerding, which is most informative and contains a further allusion to the necessity for a periodical journal (p. 29).

20. Journal of Bone and Joint Surgery, Vol. 30 B, No. 4, Nov. 1948, p. 580. Comment to the Editor.

21. Amsterdam is the city of Rembrandt Van Rijn (1606–1669), the famous Dutch painter, and the best known of his paintings are to be seen in the Rijksmuseum, notably the "Night Watch", and "The Anatomy Lesson of Dr. Tulp", which dates from 1632 and represents a dissection by Claes Pierszoon Tulp (1599–1674), known to posterity as Tulpius, a physician who was also mayor of the city.

22. The Stedelijk Museum *(municipal museum)* is more modern, and contains the most beautiful collection of Van Goghs. Van Gogh was a modern impressionist, well known for his life of torment, which is most clearly reflected in one of his paintings, "Self-portrait with Cut Ear".

23. Vol. 5 Procès Verbaux, rapports, discussions et communications particulières. (Proceedings, Vol. 5.) Brussels: Lielens, 1953.

24. Journal of Bone and Joint Surgery, Vol. 33 B, No. 3, August 1951, p. 477.

25. The castle of Drottningholm, not far from Stockholm, is known throughout the world for its extraordinary theatre. Opened in 1777 by King Gustav III (1746–1792), the theatre was also used for some magnificent operatic productions. The immense scenery – the only example of its kind, dating from the eighteenth century, and still in working order – and the exceptional depth of the stage, are its principal features. Gustave III himself wrote plays and libretti. For 15 years the high standard of the artists, indigenous and foreign, the lavishness of the decor and the costumes, ensured productions of outstanding beauty. Then the king was assassinated, which meant the end of the theatre. Revival and renovation had to wait until 1922, since when Drottningholm has atracted audiences from all over the world every season.
There are paintings and engravings illustrating the history of the theatre, examples of the original decor, and a very well-stocked library; and if all this has not succeeded in transporting the visitor back into the eighteenth century, then he needs only take his seat in the theatre, and the sight of the musicians dressed in rococo style is guaranteed to do so...
The Town Hall of Stockholm is famed for its tower, 106 metres high, and its red brick façade. Designed by Ragner Ostberg, the building was opened in 1923. It was in the great festival hall that the ceremony conferring the hat of 'Doctor of the University' used to take place (the ceremony took place for the last time in 1969).

26. Vol. 6 "Procès Verbaux, rapports, discussions et communications particulières". (Proceedings, Vol. 6.) Brussels: Lielens, 1955.

27. Journal of Bone and Joint Surgery, Vol. 36 B, No. 4, Nov. 1954, pp. 684–699.
p. 698: At the general Assembly, Professor Bryan McFarland, British Delegate, asked Sir Harry Platt to accept on behalf of the Society a Badge of office given by the British

members as a mark of their interest in the Society and their faith in its future. Sir HARRY PLATT formally acknowledged the Badge, and, after wearing it a few minutes, he placed it with a graceful acknowledgement round the neck of the President of the Congress, Dr. ETIENNE SORREL.

This is the ending of the account in the J.B.J.S. It was followed by another minor incident, however, which I feel is a typical illustration of noble spirit of the leaders of S.I.C.O.T. No sooner had the badge been conferred on E. SORREL, as recounted above, than he was invited to withdraw from the hall with JEAN DELCHEF, since their two names had been put forward for the presidency of the society. It was Jean Delchef who was elected, and without a trace of illfeeling, E. SORREL gave up the presidential badge to him. (Communication from JEAN DELCHEF, Jr.) Another point worth mentioning is that the presidential badge had been planned since 1948 by H. W. MEYERDING (see note 18, p. 72). At the Amsterdam congress in 1948, Jean Delchef, who was Secretary General at the time, said to H. W. Meyerding, President of the Congress, "We have the seal for the Society which you designed; it is to you that we owe the medal and the diploma." It was the task of the English members to carry out this project, in the circumstances we have just recalled.

28. Ibid: „Dr. DELCHEF was chosen as the first Secretary General of the Society when it was launched in Paris in 1929, and from the beginning he placed at its disposal accomodation for its documents, and the services of his own secretary. Thus for a quarter of a century he has been the mainstay of S.I.C.O.T.; indeed, as Professor BRYAN MCFARLAND said at the meeting at Berne – "but for Dr. DELCHEF the Society might well have died". The archives of the Society now fill two rooms in Dr. DELCHEF's house; and for him, S.I.C.O.T. has been, as he often said, "une affaire de famille". Members of the International Committee will remember how the intimate atmosphere of its meetings has often been enhanced by the presence of Dr. DELCHEF's young daughter and son mobilised for action – distributing ballot papers, writing on the blackboard, and making themselves generally useful". H.P.

The initials are of course those of Sir HARRY PLATT. (p. 684)

29. Vol. 7, Procès verbaux, rapports, discussions et communications particulières. (Proceedings, Vol. 7.) Brussels: Lielens, 1958. *N.B.* First support by C.I.O.M.S.

30. *Journal of Bone and Joint Surgery,* Vol. 40 B, No. 1, Feb. 1958, pp. 153–160. Exact number of participants: 636.

31. The Mountain of Montjuich is to the South East of Barcelona and towers above a vast complex of old buildings used for the 1929 International Fair, the Great Fountain, one of the tourist attractions of the town, and further on the high, round domes of the Palacio Nacional, which still houses the art treasures of the Art Museum of Catalonia. Further towards the sea, the Castillo de Montjuich is to be found, a relic of past splendour.

32. The Barrio Gotico is an impressive testimony to Barcelona's Roman and Gothic past. The ramparts *(Murallas)* are still standing, with their four fine towers; further on, the haughty and noble facade of the Palacio Episcopal, dating from the eighteenth century; and still further, the little baroque palace of San Felipe de Neri. Some other Roman fortifications have been supplanted by the Casa del Arcediano (Archdeacon's house), which nowadays houses the city's archives. Finally you come upon the cathedral, a masterpiece of Mediterranean Gothic. Not far from the cathedral are the steps leading to the Capilla de Santa Agueda, a

gothic church which is part of the Palacio Real Mayor, where Christopher Columbus presented hitherto unknown merchandise to the Catholic Kings on his return from his first voyage, and also some Red Idians, who were baptised in the cathedral.

33. Vol. 8, Rapports, discussions et communications particulières. (Proceedings, Vol. 8.) Brussels: Imprimerie des Sciences, 1961.

34. Journal of Bone and Joint Surgery, Vol. 43 B, No. 1, Feb. 1961, p. 193.

35. Pygmalion, the legendary Cypriot sculptor, fell in love with the statue of Galatea, his own work, and according to the legend persuaded Aphrodite to bring it to life. George BERNARD SHAW (1856–1950), the famous Irish dramatist, known as GBS, was inspired by this to write a play called "Pygmalion". Everyone knows the marvellous tale of ELIZA DOOLITTLE and the countless subtleties expounded by Mr. HIGGINS and Colonel PICKERING on the subject of accent and local nuance in the English language: "I'm waiting you, I'm wanting, I'm willing you". The operatic librettists made out of this one of their greatest and longestlived world successes: "My Fair Lady".

36. The Hotel Astor was one of the oldest in New York, situated on the west side of Manhattan, between 44th and 45th Street, close to Times Square. It was demolished in 1968 and has been replaced by an office block.

37. 9ᵉ Congrès International. Symposiums et Communications particulières. (Proceedings, Vol. 9.) Published by A. Bailleux, Brussels: Imprimerie des Sciences, 1964.

38. After the fall of Napoleon, the "Final Act" was signed at the Hofburg on 9 June 1815 by the most eminent diplomats of the time, to finalise the redistribution of Europe.

39. The Hofburg or Imperial Palace is a vast complex of monuments, the most ancient part dating from 1279. New wings were added between 1440 and 1913, varying according to the styles of the different periods of architecture. There you may see the Imperial Palace with the State Apartments, the secular and ecclesiastical treasuries, the Palace Chapel, home of the Vienna Boys' Choir (Wienersängerknaben), the Festival Hall, and the Spanish School of Equitation (see note 41). The magnificent building of the National Library is also part of the complex. In the so-called LEOPOLD I wing (1666) the President of the Republic and his chancellors have their offices. The Neue Hofburg (1881–1913) houses the Museum of Ethnology, the most valuable collection of arms in the world, a collection of old musical instruments, and the modern congress halls.

40. International Committee of Munich (1962). The International Committee of the Vienna Congress: W. BLOUNT: At the meeting of the International Committee in Munich, in 1962, it was suggested that it would be appropriate to have a medal offered to the President, the chairman of the Congress as well as to the President of the Society. It was agreed last September that the United States's Chapter of S.I.C.O.T. should supply such a medal; since then the medal has been prepared. I now want to deliver it to you, Mr. CORNET, as Treasurer of the Society, and I think it is particularly fitting that the first to receive this medal should be

120

the distinguished Colleague from the United States, our good friend PHILIP WILSON, and I charge the President HACKENBROCH with the responsibility of making the presentation at the First General Assembly of the Société Internationale. (S.I.C.O.T. archives.)

41. The Spanische Reitschule *(Spanish School of Equitation)* is a curiosity typical of Vienna. It was founded in 1580; the style of equitation perfected in Vienna by de Pluvinel, riding instructor to LOUIS XIII (1601–1643) has hardly changed since those times. The horses are pure-bred Lippizaners.

42. The Versailles of Austria, the incomparable Castle of Schoenbrunn is linked with the history of the Hapsburgs. Napoleon concluded the peace treaty of Schoenbrunn in 1809. His son, l'Aiglon or Duc de Reichstadt, was exiled there, where he died at the age of 21. FRANZ JOSEF I, the Well-Beloved (1830–1916), the romantic husband of the Empress ELISABETH (1837–1898), better known as SISSI, was born and died there. The Hall of Mirrors at Schoenbrunn is almost as splendid as that of Versailles.

43. The Staatsoper is a world centre of classical and operatic music. Dating from the beginning of the last century, it was demolished during the Second World War, and completely reconstructed in all its former magnificence. It is necessary to book 12–18 months in advance, and it was a considerable feat on the part of the Viennese Committee to succeed in the booking the Vienna Opera House for S.I.C.O.T..

44. 10e Congrès. Symposia, discussions, conférences et communications particulières. (Proceedings, Vol. 10.) Published by Jean Delchef, Jr. Brussels: Acta Medica Belgica, 1967.

45. The Museum of French Monuments is part of the Palais de Chaillot, on one of the most beautiful esplanades in Paris. Apart from some beautiful examples of French sculpture, there are many sketches, designs and schemes illustrating the initial stages (plans, draughts) of the building and construction of the most important French monuments.

46. The Cluny Museum is built on the site of the "Thermal baths of Lutèce" or the "Thermal baths of Julien", which were partly excavated in 1946. The remains are impressive: baths, frigidarium, vaulted hall, etc. After changing hands a great many times, this imposing Gallo-Roman complex became the property of the monks of Cluny, who added a hall of residence which was confiscated during the French Revolution. Later the buildings passed into the judicious ownership of ALEXANDRE DE SOMMERARD, whose collections, continuously added to and improved, and nowadays consisting of some 23,000 items, were given the status of National Monument. One of the most beautiful exhibits is the group of six tapestries, "La Dame à la Licorne".

47. One of the finest buildings in Paris, and still called the Palais Garnier after the architect, CHARLES GARNIER (1825–1898) who supervised the building between 1862 and 1874. As for Carmen, everyone knows of the cigar maker's tumultuous love affairs, which inspired GEORGES BIZET (1838–1875).

48. LOUIS LE VAU (1612–1670), famous French architect who designed the Louvre, the Tuileries and the Chateau of Vaux-le-Vicomte. He was responsible for the design of the buildings of Versailles, which were completed by Jules Hardouin-Mansart (1646–1708), each detail requiring the approval of Louis XIV (1643–1715) himself. But the vast Orangery is Le Vau's own work, access to it being by way of the Staircase of One Hundred Steps.

49. 11ᵉ Congrès, conférences, symposia et communications particulières. (Proceedings, Vol. 11.) JEAN DELCHEF, Jr. (ed.). Brussels: Imprimerie des Sciences, 1970.

50. It was in 1521 that the last Aztec emperor, Cuahtemoc, surrendered at Tenochtitlan, the last town to be conquered by the sword and fire of the Spanish.

51. All Mexican towns have a more or less central square, in the middle of which, intially, some statue was to be erected on a pedestal or *zocalo*. More often than not the statue never arrived, but the *zocalo* remained as it was, or became the Plaza Mayor. In Mexico City the Zocalo is the site of the cathedral, which was built on the ruins of an Aztec temple. It was begun in 1573 and not finished until the last century; it is the most beautiful and important monument of religious architecture in the Americas, and comprises examples of three centuries' architecture.
Chapultepec: one of the oldest natural parks in the Americas. Within its confines ist the castle of the same name, built in the last century as the residence of the unfortunate Emperor MAXIMILIAN of Austria (1832–1867) who was also briefly Emperor of Mexico.
Parque de Alameda: the very beautiful central park, dating from the beginning of this century, a fine place for walking and relaxing.
The Anthropological Museum: a monument erected to the glory of the cultures of the pre-Columbus and pre-Cortès eras. There are 25 rooms of exhibits and numerous other aids to study. Mexico has about 11,000 archaeological sites.

52. Palacio de Bellas Artes *(Palace of Fine Arts)* – the home of the Ballet Folclorico. This spectacle, and the "Deer Dance" in particular, is unforgettable.

53. Fifty kilometres to the North of Mexico City, Teotihuacan, 'city of the gods', is an immense city of several tens of square kilometres. It is dominated by the famous Pyramids of the Sun and Moon, and the Temple of Quetzalcoatl, the plumed serpent.

54. Seventy-five kilometres to the North of Mexico City is the site of Tepozotlan, with its baroque church in the Churrigueresque style of the eighteenth century, with its 300 sculptures on the facade and the most magnificent reredos in New Spain.

55. 12ᵉ Congrès. (Proceedings, Vol. 12.) JEAN DELCHEF, Jr., R. DE MARNEFFE and E. VANDER ELST (eds.). Amsterdam: Excerpta Medica, 1974.

56. The heavy losses resulting from the attack in Munich: 17 dead (11 Israeli athletes, 5 Palestinians and a West German policeman). 5 September 1972.

57. Thanks to the generosity of a patron of the arts, FREDERIC MANN, this auditorium has exceptionally good acoustics. It is a world centre for classical music.

58. Caesarea, about 20 km to the North of Tel Aviv, on the coast. HEROD the Great built the town between 28 and 14 B.C., and provided it with a port which is famous for its lighthouse; with ramparts, with several white marble palaces, an aqueduct and a theatre.

Vespasien was crowned Emperor there, and the ruins, which may still be seen today, are of great interest to the historian. Herod gave the town its name in honour of the emperor Augustus.

59. Massada, a rock on the edge of the Judea desert, towers 400 metres above the Dead Sea. It is here that one of the most dramatic episodes in the history of the Jewish people took place. The Romans dominated this region from the 1st century B.C., and King Herod the Great (73-4 B.C.) had a fortress built there with casemates, battlements, arsenals, etc. ... but there was another important detail: there were reservoirs for the fresh water which was very providently brought into the area via underground conduits. In the year 66, a group of rebel Jews, or Zealots, attacked and seized the fortress, dislodging the Roman garrison. In the year 72, Flavius Silva decided to take back this island of resistance, and besieged Massada. At the foot of the rock he had a high wall built to surround and cut off any retreating soldiers, and a ramp of earth and stone was erected leading up to the wall. After a long siege, the rebels saw that there was no hope. One night the chief of the Zealots decided that they should die gloriously rather than survive in slavery. He ordered a few of his men to slaughter the 960 men, women and children who had all accepted this tragic fate. When the Romans arrived they were greeted by a profound silence.
A Roman officer, Flavius Joseph (37–100) wrote an account of this, and may be considered as one of the first 'reporters'. Yigael Yadin, the well-known archaeologist, has made it his task to look after the site and has made a number of most interesting discoveries.

60. Founded in 1479 by King Christian I (1426–1481) and progressively developed until 1728, the year in which the University of Copenhagen was destroyed by the fire which ravaged the town. The buildings of the university were once more razed to the ground in 1807 by the English bombardment during the Napoleonic wars. The present buildings date from the period of the reconstruction that followed this, and are a fine example of the neo-gothic style. Two points of interest: the entrance hall is decorated with motifs inspired by Pompéi, and in the courtyard there is a small medieval building dating from around 1420, the oldest of its type inside the ancient ramparts. Nowadays it is here that the Council of the University meets.

61. The Town Hall of Copenhagen, built between 1892 and 1905, was designed to be the place where every citizen could feel "at home". To this end there is the great festival hall, with a "Mediterranean" atmosphere; it is immense and colourful and reminiscent of a piazza. There is also a tower, 105 metres in height, and the cosmic clock designed by Jens Olsen near the entrance.

62. Just as famous as the Little Mermaid (Den Lille Havfrue) is the pleasure park of Tivoli, which dates from 1843. During the summer there are no less than 35,000 visitors each day, who go to enjoy the multitude of diversions it affords. It is at the same time a botanical garden and a cultural centre, with concert halls, etc.

63. Built by Christian IV (1577–1648), the 'builder King', the castle of Frederiksborg was destroyed by fire in 1850. The great chapel, with its organs dating from 1610, and the Gateway of the Mint, and the buildings surrounding the delightful S-shaped bridge, all survived the fire. It is now the wealthiest museum in Denmark.

123

64. Fredensborg, in the North of Zeeland, is the summer residence of the Danish Royal Family. The earliest buildings date from 1720.

The castle of Kronborg, at Elsinore (Helsingor in Danish) was made famous by W. SHAKESPEARE (1563–1616), who set his play *Hamlet* there ("To be or not to be..."). The castle is about 1000 years old.

65. The Vikings were Scandinavian plunderers who made expeditions on all the seas of Europe. With nothing but their light vessels, which carried from four to eighty men, they reached Spain in 844, Italy in 860, Ireland in 840, went back up the Seine to Paris in 844–885, and ruled Normandy until 911. At the same time they invaded most of England and the Frisian Islands (850–875) and even went as far as Constantinople in 865.

According to local lore, the wreckage of a Viking ship lay in the Fjord of Roskilde. During the summer of 1962, five wrecks were found, and carefully preserved and reconstructed after a great deal of hard work. Subsequently a museum of archaeology was built on the site of this exceptional find, and it is now a centre of scientific progress in archaeology.

66. The cathedral of Roskilde is a group of red brick buildings dating back to the eleventh century, and has been the site of burial of the kings of Denmark throughout the last six centuries.

67. Grundtvigskirchen, the finest example of the transformation of a Danish country church into a modern cathedral. It was constructed from 1921 to 1940.

68. The Ballet of the Theatre Royal of Copenhagen was founded in 1772 and directed by a succession of Italian and French ballet masters. The great story-teller HANS CHRISTIAN ANDERSEN almost made his début on stage there.

V. Those Who Made S.I.C.O.T.

«La reconnaissance est la mémoire du cœur»
(Unknown Author)

1. I have not been lucky enough to find photographs of all these great men of our field, despite a great deal of research and correspondence, and I ask the reader to bear with me.

2. At the beginning, the distinction between President of the Society and President of the Congress was not altogether clear. For example, Sir Robert Jones was not a founder, but was first President of the Society and President of the first Congress. W. MURK-JANSEN was a founder and was second President of the Society. Louis OMBREDANNE was a founder and President of the Society; VITTORIO PUTTI was a founder and President of a Congress; JEAN DELCHEF was a founder, Secretary General from 1929 to 1954, and President of the Society from 1954 to 1960. ROBERT MERLE D'AUBIGNÉ was President of a Congress and President of the Society. Taking all this into account, I have tried to give all concerned their appropriate place. I have also included ANTOINE BAILLEUX, who was Secretary General from 1954 to 1966, CHARLES PARISEL, Treasurer from 1945 to 1957, and JOSEPH CORNET, Treasurer from 1957 to 1966.

3. At the end of each of the three sections there is a list of bio-bibliographic references.

N.B. I regret that I have been unable to include the Vice-Presidents of the Society in this section. I would, however, like at this juncture to express the gratitude we all owe to them. At the same time I would like to thank all those who, by their faithful and regular attendance at congresses, ensured the viability of S.I.C.O.T. They too 'made' S.I.C.O.T.

A. The Founders

I.   PHILIP ERLACHER
II.   HANS SPITZY 1872–1956
III.   JEAN DELCHEF 1882–1962
IV.   PAUL LORTHIOIR
V.   ADOLPHE MAFFEI 1872–1945
VI.   RAMON SAN RICART 1882–1956
VII.   FRED ALBEE 1875–1945
VIII. WILLIAM BAER 1872–1931
IX.   HENRY W. MEYERDING 1884–1969
X.   LOUIS OMBREDANNE 1871–1956
XI.   LOUIS ROCHER 1876–1957
XII.   ETIENNE SORREL 1882–1965
XIII. Sir THOMAS A. T. FAIRBANK 1876–1961
XIV.   RICCARDO GALEAZZI 1886–1952
XV.   VITTORIO PUTTI 1880–1940
XVI.   WILLEM MURK JANSEN 1867–1935
XVII. JEAN JIANO   –1971
XVIII. PATRICK HAGLUND 1870–1937
XIX.   HENNING WALDENSTRÖM 1877–1971
XX.   ALFRED MACHARD 1871–1931
XXI.   JAN ZAHRADNICEK 1882–1958

XXII. ANTOINE BAILLEUX, Secretary General 1954–1966
XXIII. CHARLES PARISEL (1878–1963), Treasurer 1945–1957
XXIV. JOSEPH CORNET (–1966), Treasurer 1957–1966

126

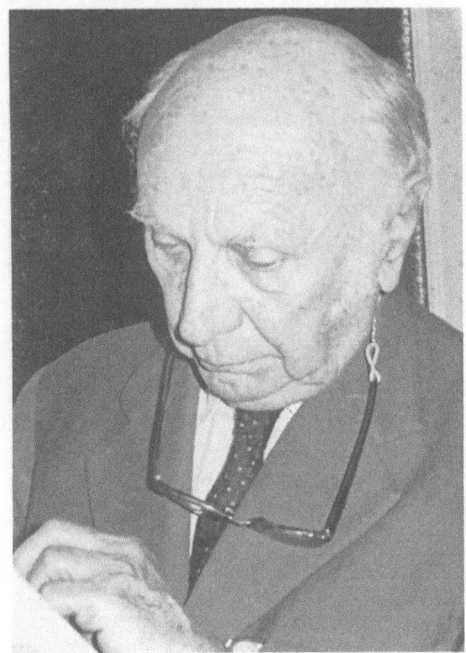

Philip Erlacher

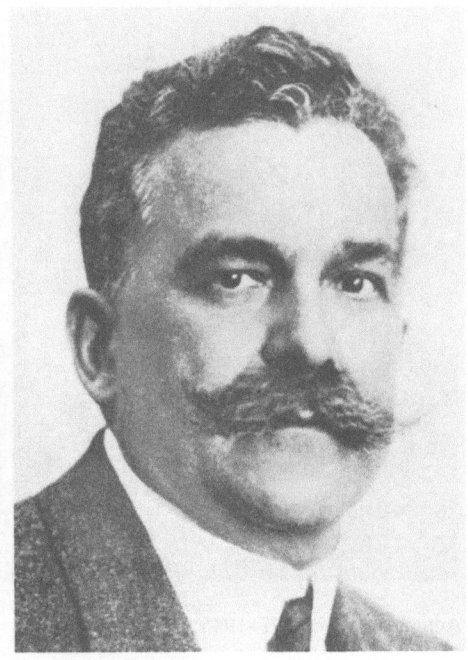

Hans Spitzy (1872–1956)

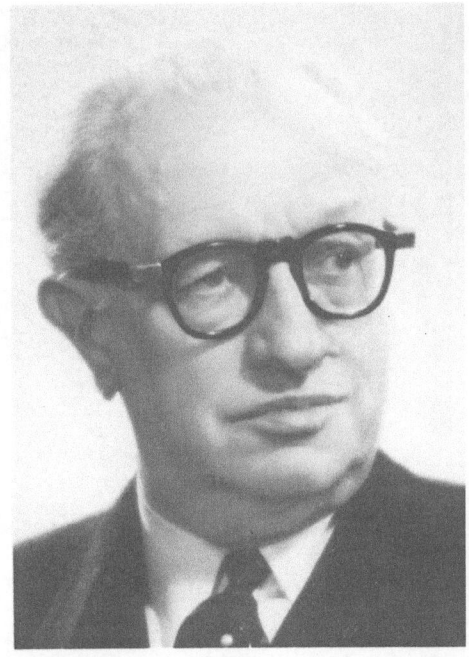

Jean Delchef (1882–1962)

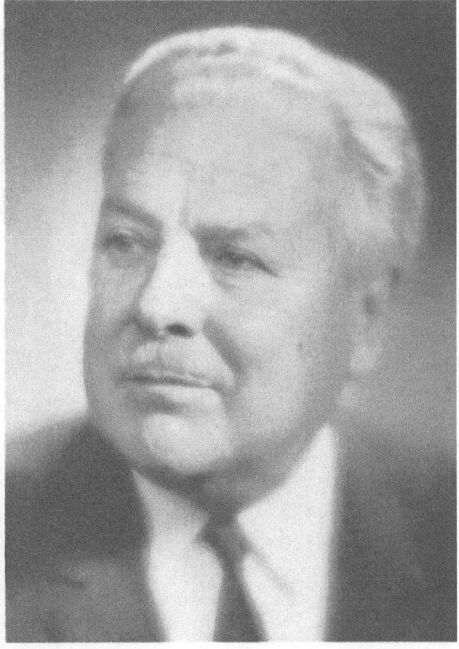

Paul Lorthioir

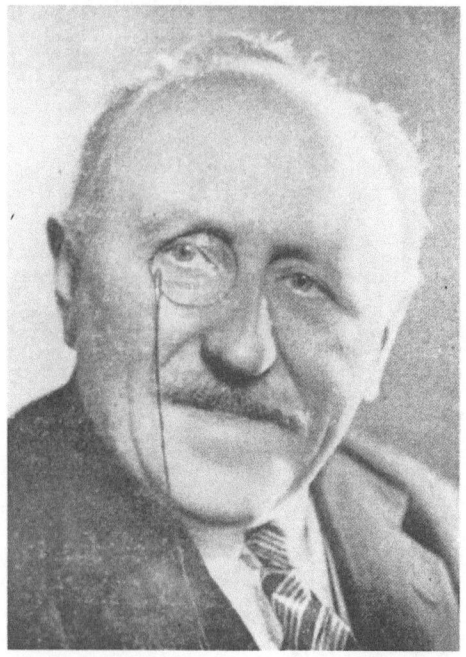
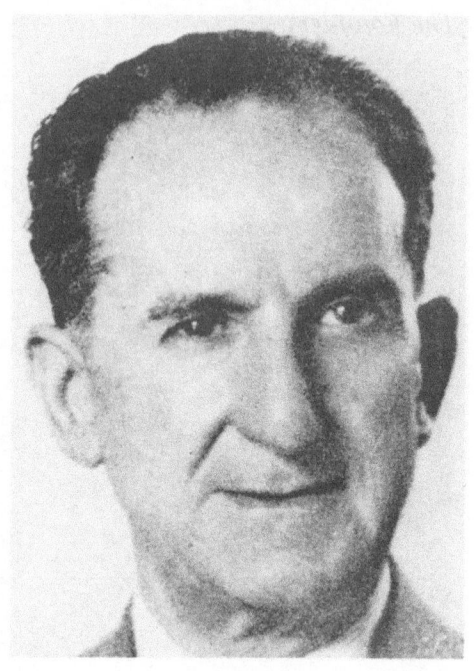

Adolphe Maffei (1872–1945)   Ramon San Ricart (1882–1956)

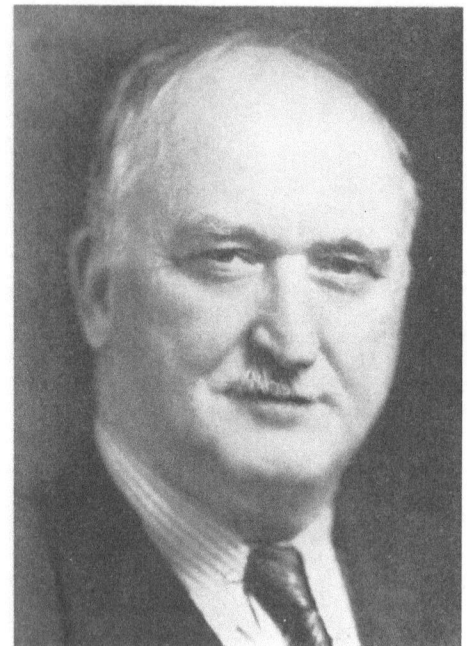
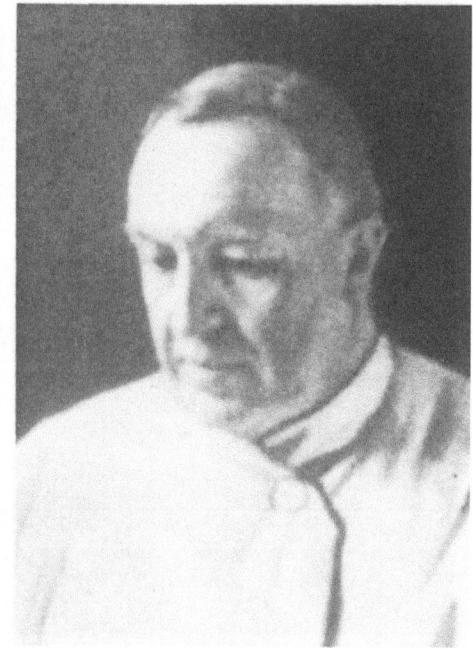

Fred Albee (1875–1945)   William Baer (1872–1931)

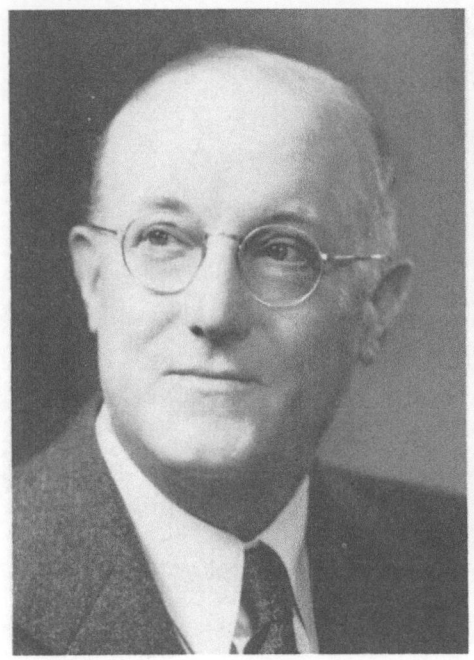
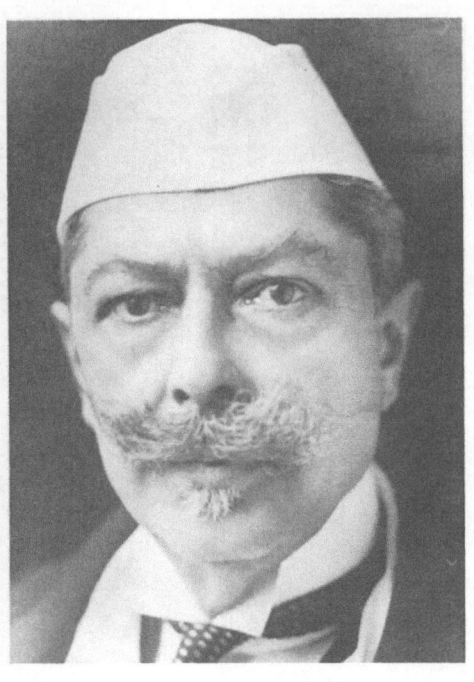

Henry W. Meyerding (1884–1969)   Louis Ombredanne (1871–1956)

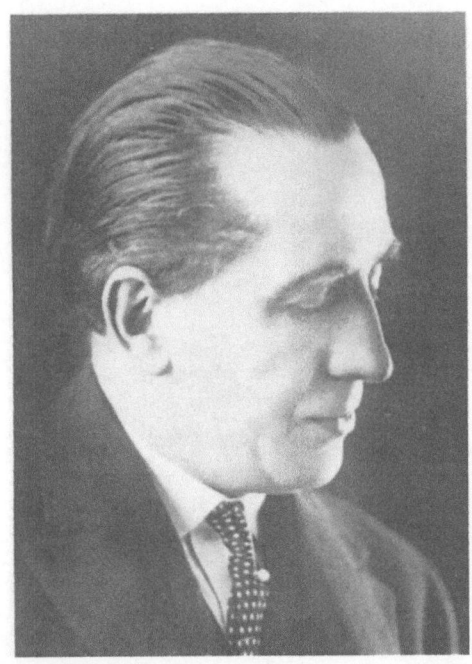
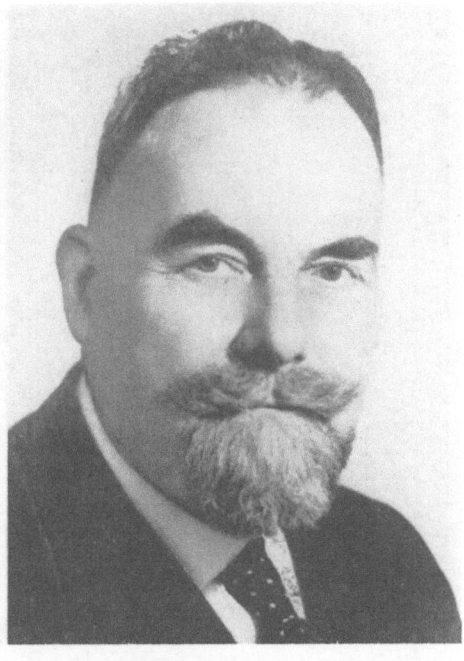

Louis Rocher (1876–1957)   Etienne Sorrel (1882–1965)

129

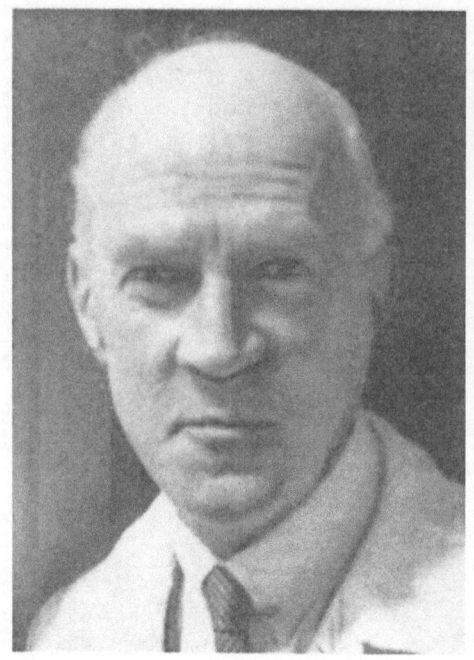

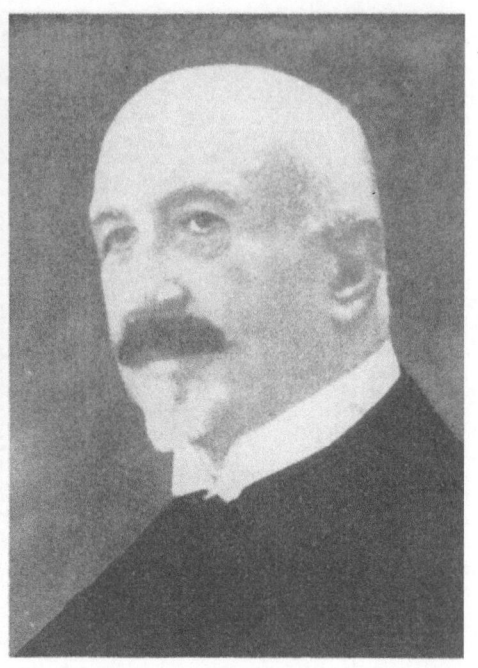

Sir Thomas A. T. Fairbank (1876–1961)   Riccardo Galeazzi (1886–1952)

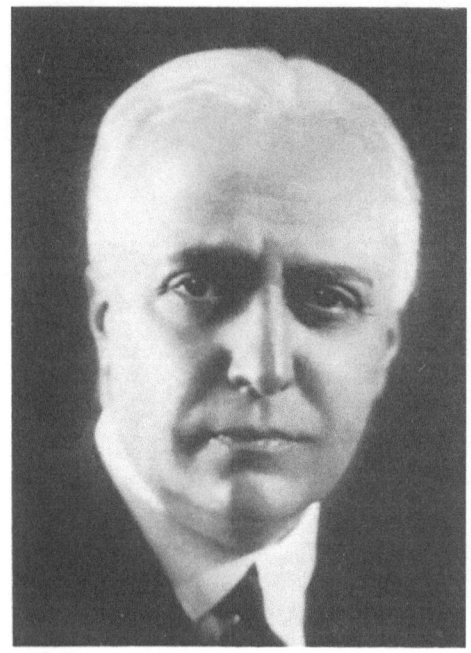

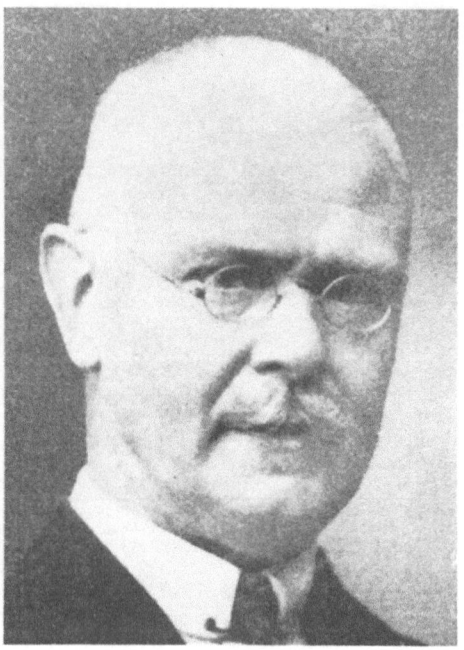

Vittorio Putti (1880–1940)   Willem Murk Jansen (1867–1935)

130

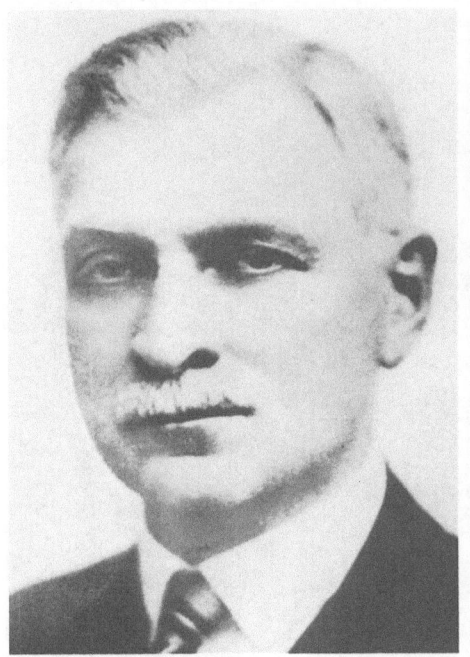

Jean Jiano (–1971)

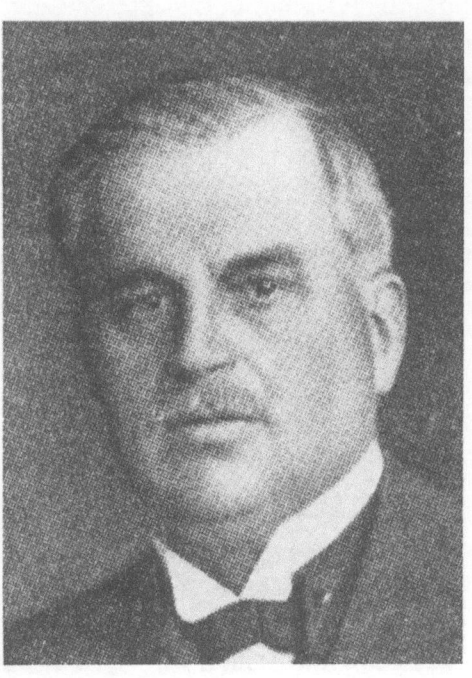

Patrick Haglund (1870–1937)

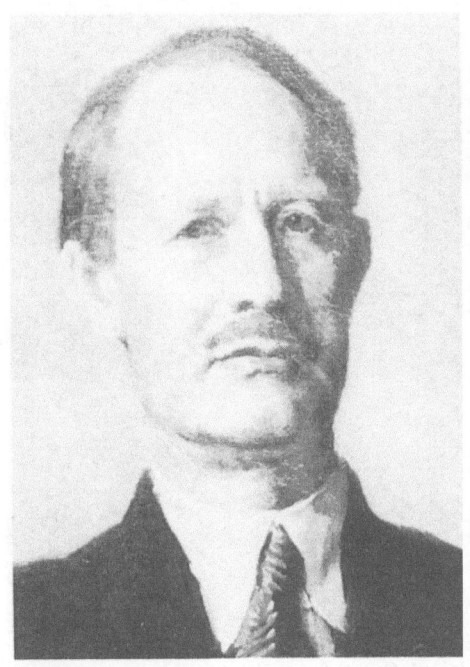

Henning Waldenström (1877–1971)

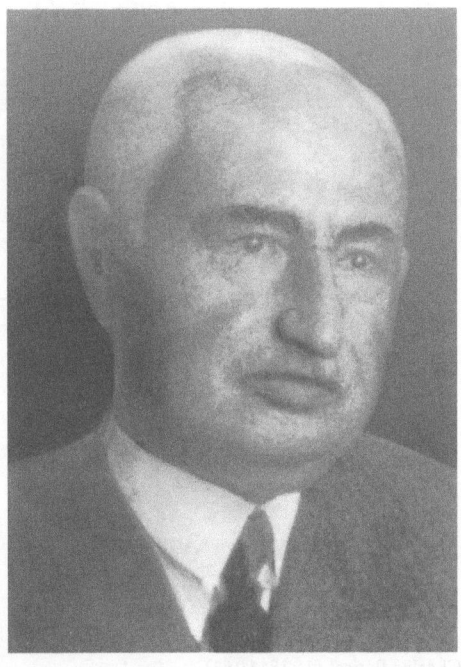

Alfred Machard (1871–1931)

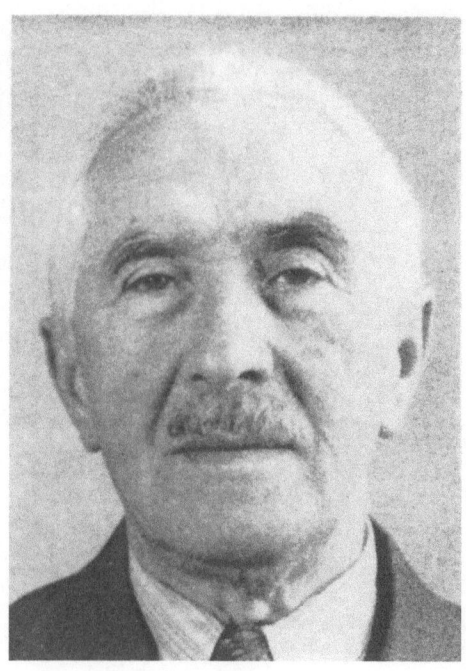

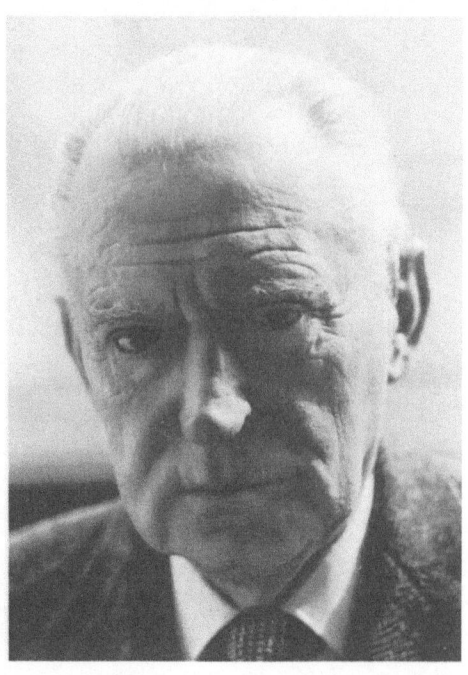

Jean Zahradnicek (1882–1958)
Reproduced with kind permission of J.B.J.S.

Antoine Bailleux, Secretary General (1954–1966)

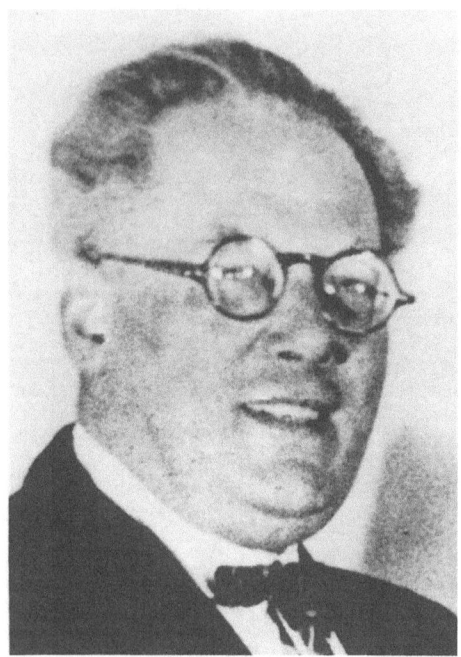

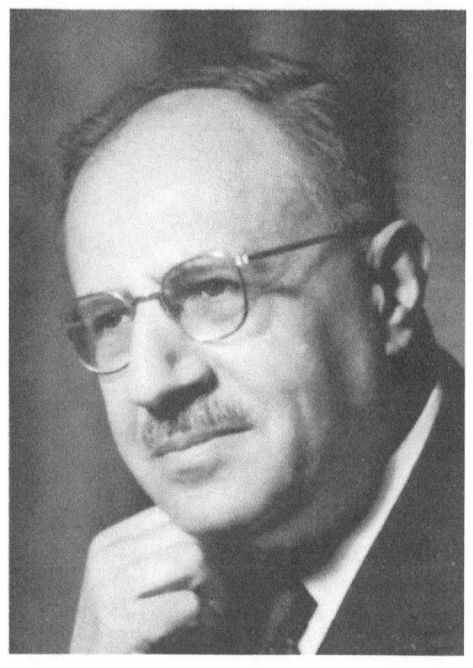

Charles Parisel (1878–1963),
Treasurer (1945–1957)

Joseph Cornet (–1966),
Treasurer (1957–1966)

132

HANS SPITZY: Proceedings of the Barcelona Congress (note 29), p. 68.

JEAN DELCHEF: *Journal of Bone and Joint Surgey,* Vol. 44 B, No. 4, British Volume, Nov. 1962.

ADOLPHE MAFFEI: Brussels Meeting (note 17), p. 18.

RAMON SAN RICART: Proceedings of the Barcelona Congress (note 29), p. 78.

FRED ALBEE: Proceedings of the London Congress (note 9), p. 37.

WILLIAM BAER: Proceedings of the London Congress (note 9), p. 37.

HENRY W. MEYERDING: *Journal of Bone and Joint Surgery.* Vol. 32 B, No. 4, Nov. 1950, p. 493.

N. B. Under the heading "Historical Reviews" there are many references to all the great men of Anglo-Saxon orthopaedic surgery and traumatology.

LOUIS OMBREDANNE: Proceedings of the Barcelona Congress (note 29), p. 59. La Presse Médicale, 65th year, No. 5, pp. 99–100.

LOUIS ROCHER: Revue de Chirurgie Orthopédique, Vol. 43, Nos. 5 and 6, 1957.

ETIENNE SORREL: Presse Médicale, 1965, No. 53.

Sir THOMAS A. T. FAIRBANK: *Journal of Bone and Joint Surgery,* THOMAS FAIRBANK Birthday Volume, Vol. 38 B, No. 1, Feb. 1956.

RICCARDO GALEAZZI: Proceedings of the Bern Congress (note 26), p. 94.

VITTORIO PUTTI: Proceedings of the Brussels Meeting (note 27), p. 15. *Journal of Bone and Joint Surgerey,* Vol. 39 B, No. 2, May 1957, pp. 423–425.

WILLEM MURK JANSEN: Proceedings of the Bologna-Rome Congress (note 13), p. 37. Archivum Chirurgicum Neerlandicum, Vol. II, Fasc. 4, 1950.

JEAN JIANO (reminder).

PATRICK HAGLUND: Proceedings of the Brussels Meeting (note 27), p. 85.

HENNING WALDENSTRÖM: *Journal of Bone and Joint Surgery,* Vol. 34 B, No. 3, Aug. 1952, p. 529.

ALFRED MACHARD: Proceedings of the London Congress (note 9), p. 44. Geschichte der Schweizerischen Gesellschaft für Orthopaedie. Hans Debrunner. Bern: Buchdruckerei Paul Haupt, AG.

JAN ZAHRADNICEK: *Journal of Bone and Joint Surgery,* Vol. 41 A, No. 2, Mar. 1959, p. 376.

CHARLES PARISEL: *Le Scalpel,* No. 21, May 5, 1963.

JOSEPH CORNET: Acta Orthopaedica Belgica, 1966,

B. Presidents of S.I.C.O.T.

1st President:	Sir ROBERT JONES (1858–1933)	1929–1933
2nd President:	W. MURK JANSEN* (1867–1935) Founder	1933–1935
3rd President:	LOUIS OMBREDANNE* (1871–1956) Founder	1936–1951
4th President:	Sir HARRY PLATT	1951–1954
5th President:	JEAN DELCHEF* (1882–1962) Founder	1954–1960
6th President:	BRYAN MCFARLAND (–1962)	1960–1962
7th President:	MATHIAS HACKENBROCH	1962–1966
8th President:	STEN FRIBERG (1902–1977)	1966–1969
9th President:	ROBERT MERLE D'AUBIGNÉ	1969–1972
10th President:	FLOYD H. JERGESEN	1972–1975
11th President:	CALOGERO CASUCCIO	1975–1978

---

* The Founders are listed, but their photographs do not appear here (see A).

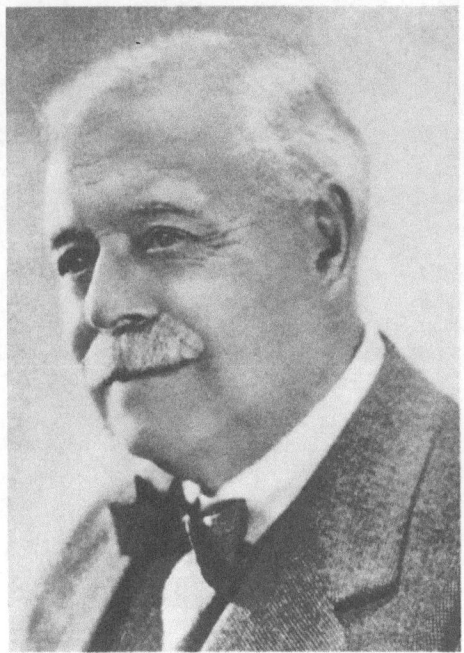

1st President (1929–1933)
Sir Robert Jones (1858–1933)

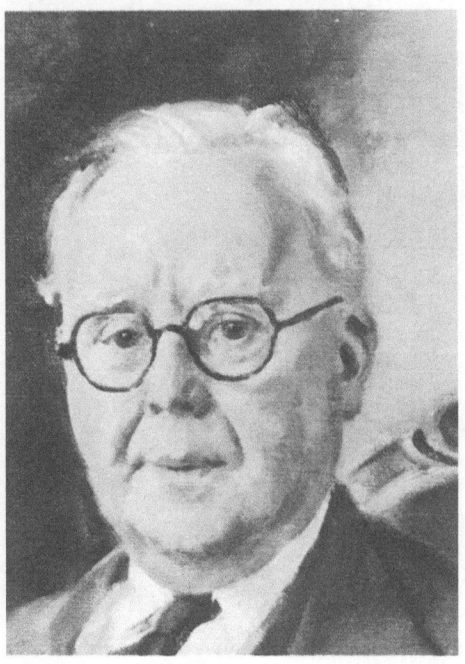

4th President (1951–1954)
Sir Harry Platt

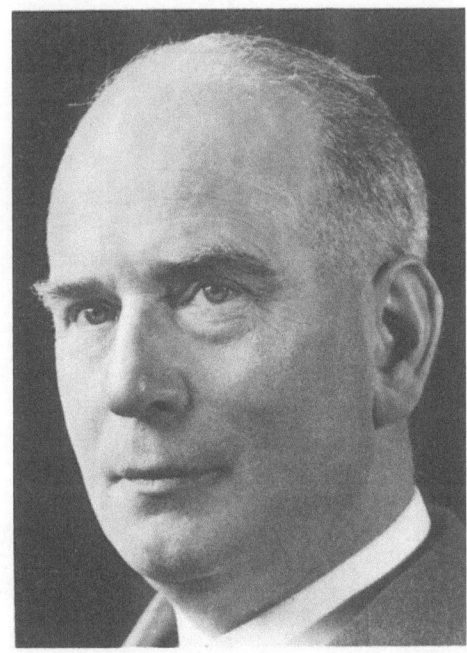

6th President (1960–1962)
Bryan McFarland (–1962)

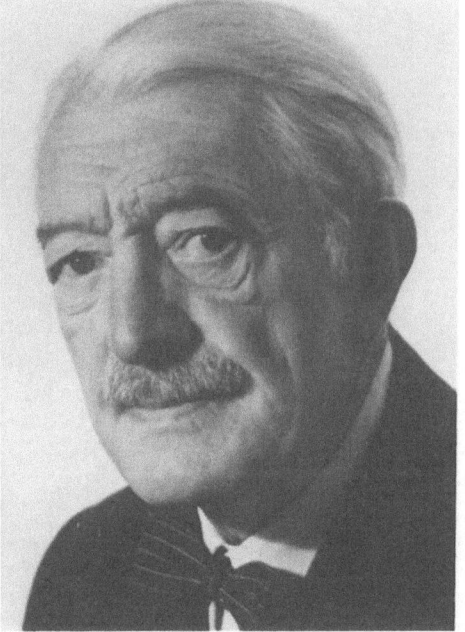

7th President (1962–1966)
Mathias Hackenbroch

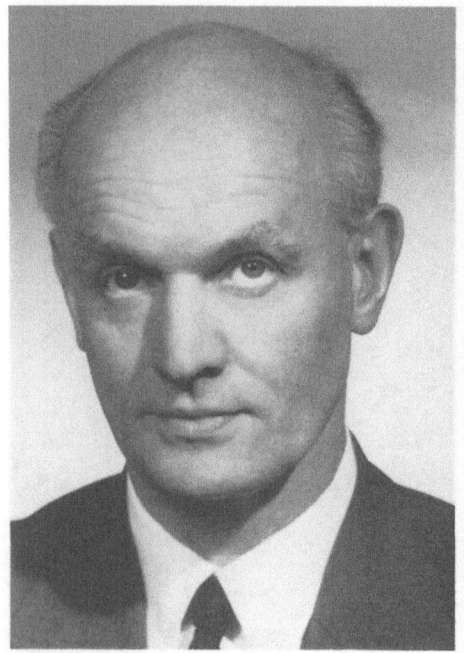
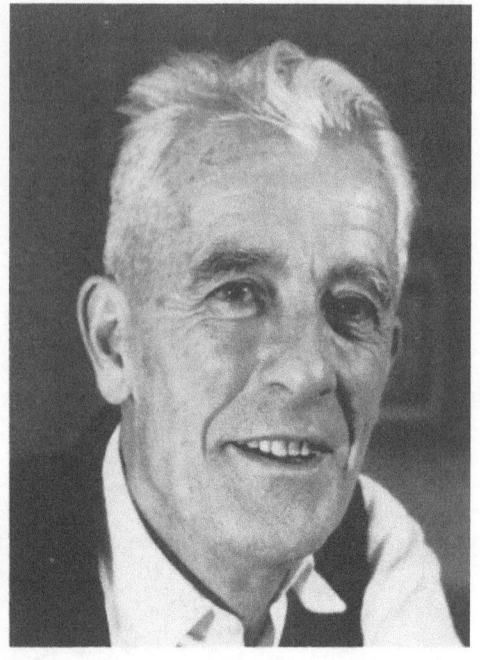

8th President (1966–1969)
Sten Friberg (1902–1977)

9th President (1969–1972)
Robert Merle d'Aubigné

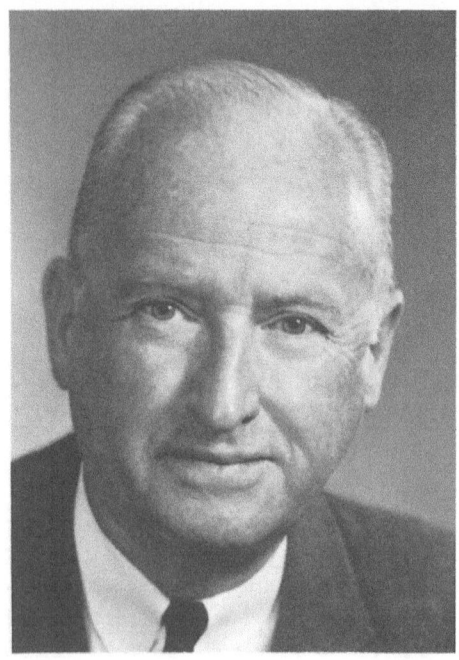
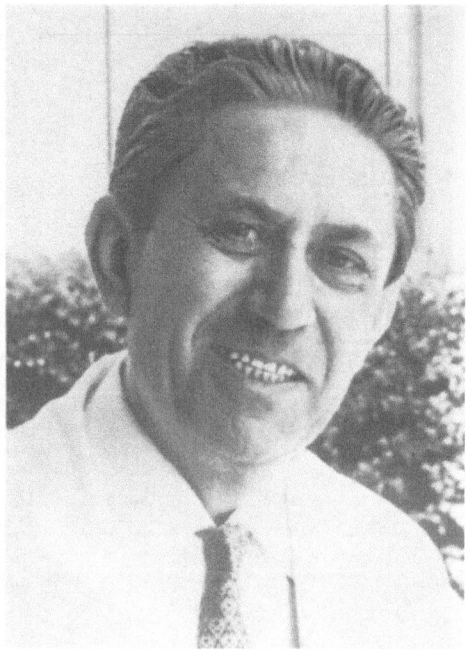

10th President (1972–1975)
Floyd H. Jergesen

11th President (1975–1978)
Calogero Casuccio

136

Bio-bibliographic References

Sir ROBERT JONES: Proceedings of the London Congress, 1933 (note 13, p. 21). G. R. GIRDLESTONE: "The Robert Jones tradition". Journal of Bone and Joint Surgery, Vol. 30 B, No. 1, Feb. 1948, pp. 187–195.

GORONWY THOMAS: From bonesetter to orthopaedic surgeon. Annals of the Royal College of Surgeons of England, Vol. 55, Sept.–Oct. 1974.

Sir HARRY PLATT: *Journal of Bone and Joint Surgerey*, Vol. 30 B, No. 1, Feb. 1948, p. 205.

BRYAN McFARLAND: *Journal of Bone and Joint Surgerey*, Vol. 33 B, No. 4, Nov. 1951, p. 642.

MATHIAS HACKENBROCH: Zum 80. Geburtstag. *Zeitschrift für Orthopaedie und ihre Grenzgebiete*, 112, No. 5, 1974.

CALOGERO CASUCCIO: La Clinica Orthopedica, Vol. 26, 1975–1976, pp. 1–6.

C. Presidents of the Congresses

Paris, 1930, President: Sir ROBERT JONES (1857–1933)*
London, 1933, President: GABRIEL NOVÉ-JOSSERAND (1868–1948)
Bologna-Rome, 1936, President: VITTORIO PUTTI (1880–1940)**
(Berlin 1939, did not take place), President: GEORG HOHMANN
Amsterdam, 1948, President: HENRY W. MEYERDING (1884–1969)**
Stockholm, 1951, Honorary President: HENNING WALDENSTRÖM (1877–1971)** President: RICHARD SCHERB (1880–1955)
Bern, 1954, Honorary President: RICHARD SCHERB President: ETIENNE SORREL (1882–1965)
Barcelona, 1957, President: JOSÉ VALLS (1896–1977)
New York, 1960, President: JOSEPH TRUETA (1897–1977)
Vienna, 1963, President: PHILIP D. WILSON: (–1969)
Paris, 1966, President: ROBERT MERLE D'AUBIGNÉ
Mexico, 1969, President: JUAN FARILL (1902–1973)
Tel Aviv-Jerusalem, President: ERNST SPIRA (1901–1976)
Copenhagen, 1975, President: KNUD JANSEN
Kyoto, 1978, President: TAMIKAZU AMAKO

---

* See B: Presidents of S.I.C.O.T.
** See A: The Founders.

Presidents of the Congresses

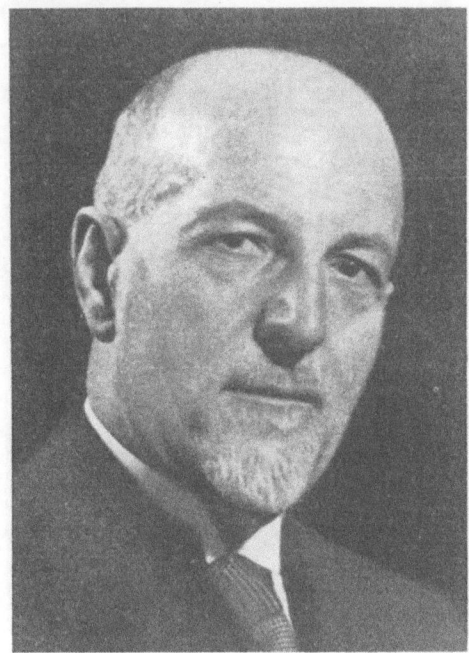

London, 1933
Gabriel Nové-Josserand

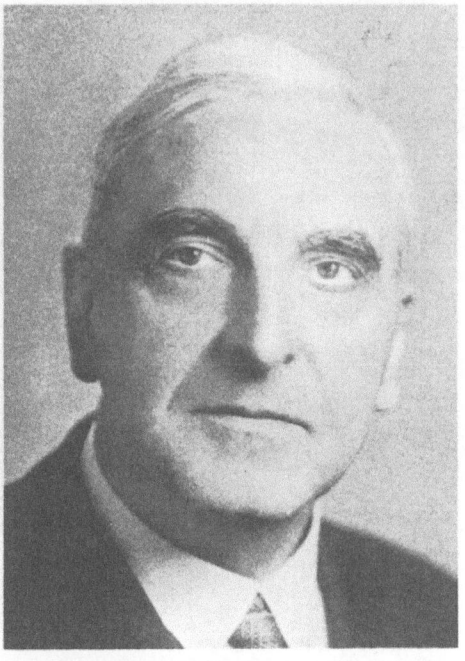

Bern, 1954, Honorary President:
Richard Scherb

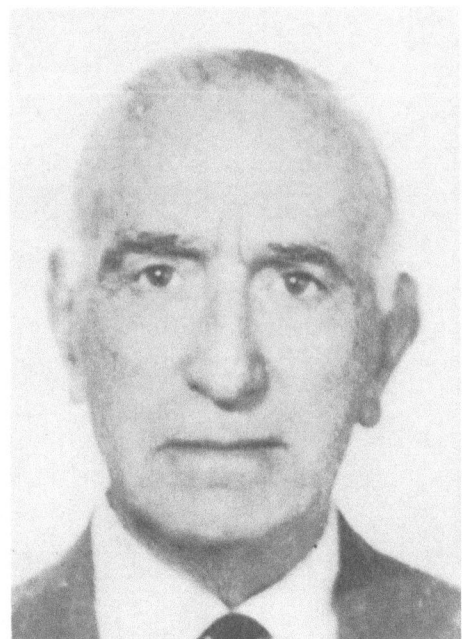

Barcelona, 1957, President:
José Valls (1896–1977)

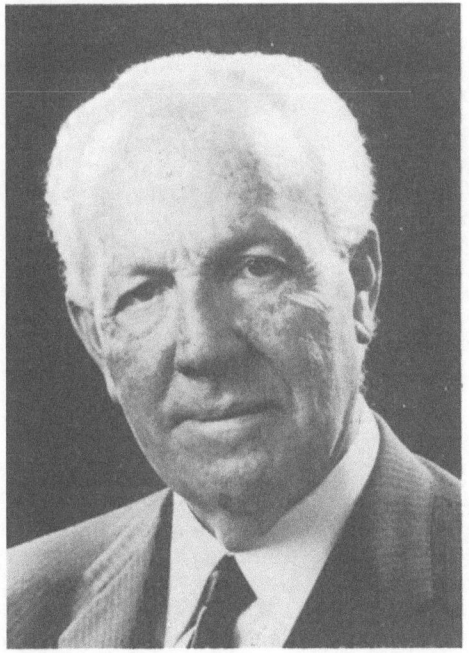

New York, 1960, President:
Joseph Trueta (–1977)

139

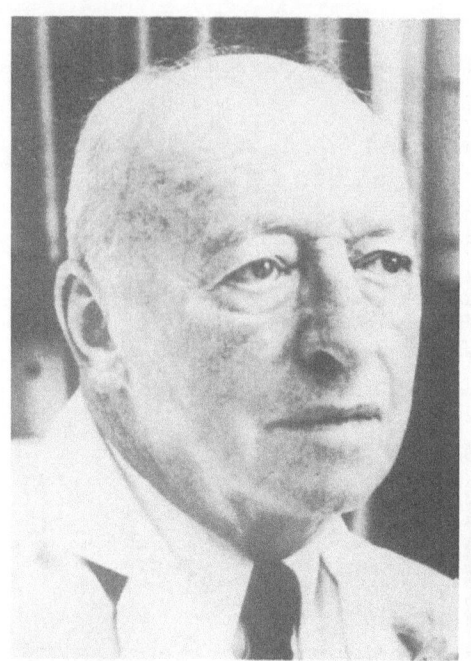

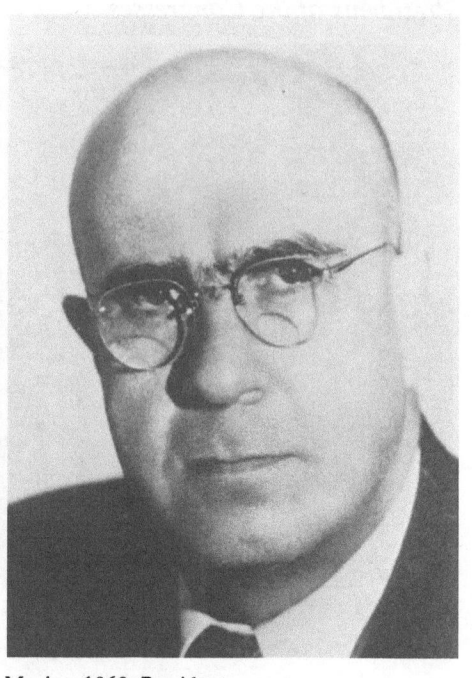

Vienna, 1963, President:
Philip D. Wilson (–1969)

Mexico, 1969, President:
Juan Farill (1902–1973)

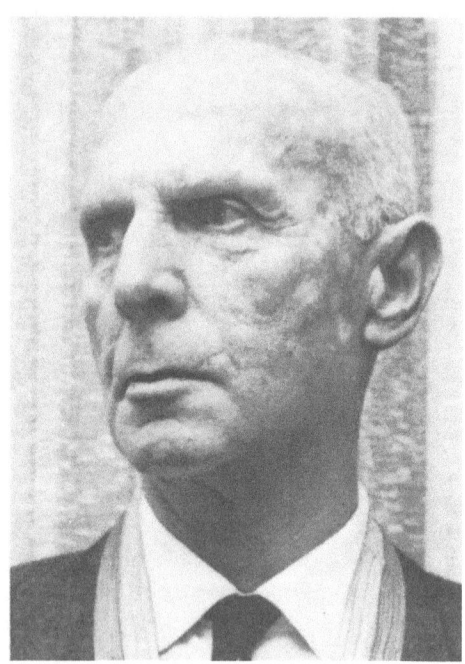

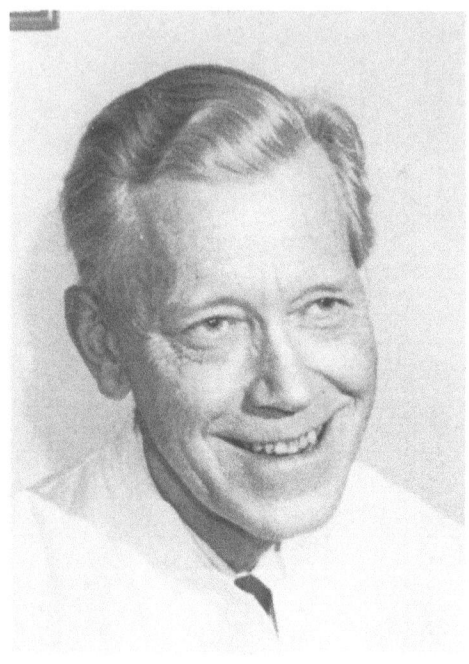

Tel Aviv-Jerusalem, President:
Ernst Spira (1901–1976)

Copenhagen, 1975, President:
Knud Jansen

140

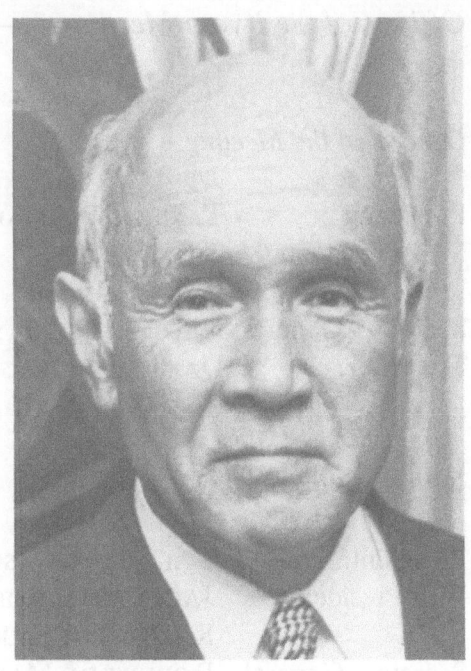

Kyoto, 1978, S.I.C.O.T.
President: Tamikazu Amako

Bio-bibliographic References to C

GABRIEL NOVÉ-JOSSERAND: Proceedings of the Stockholm Congress (note 23), p. 52.

RICHARD SCHERB: Proceedings of the Barcelona Congress (note 29), p. 115.

HANS DEBRUNNER: Geschichte der Schweizerischen Gesellschaft für Orthopaedie. Bern: Buchdruckerei Paul Haupt AG, pp. 15–16.

JOSÉ VALLS: *International Orhopaedics,* Vol. 2, No. 2

JOSEPH TRUETA: *International Orthopaedics,* Vol. 1, No. 4

PHILIP D. WILSON: *Journal of Bone and Joint Surgery,* Vol. 30 B, No. 1, Feb. 1948, pp. 205–206; also Vol. 51 A, No. 7, Oct. 1969, pp. 1445–1447.

JUAN FARILL: Anales de Orthopedia y Traumatologia, Vol. IX, Nos. 3 and 4, 1973.

ERNST SPIRA: *International Orthopaedics,* Vol. 2, No. 1. *Journal of Hand Surgery,* Vol. 2, No. 1, p. 83.

141

Officers of the Kyoto Meeting: 15–20 October 1978

Officers of the Meeting

President: TAMIKAZU AMAKO
Vice Presidents: TETSUO ITO
                     YASUTO ITAMI
Secretary General: NAOICHI TSUMAYA
Treasurer: DAIJI KASHIWAGI

Officers of the Society

President: CALOGERO CASUCCIO
Vice Presidents: JACQUES G. ROBICHON
                     KETI T. DHOLAKIA
Secretary General: ROBERT DE MARNEFFE
Treasurer: EDOUARD VANDER ELST
Editorial Secretary: JAQUES WAGNER

Envoi

"And so I bring to an end an all too inadequate tribute"* to the History of S.I.C.O.T., to the works and achievements of those who made S.I.C.O.T.

Of course I realise that this historical outline is by no means complete, and that there are a number of gaps that ought to be filled, as any critic could point out. Still I have done what I could with the material that was available to me; and the main ingredient was my own enthusiasm for S.I.C.O.T. I joined the Society in 1954 at the time of the Bern Congress. I was unable to attend the Congresses in Barcelona, New York and Vienna for a multitude of reasons for which Chance and Destiny are doubtless to blame.

Since the Paris Congress of 1966 I have had the great privilege of attending all the congresses and helping within the scope of my abilities those higher up in the ranks who work for the furtherance and progress of S.I.C.O.T. The result of this is that I have had the good fortune to know a number of the Great Men, deceased or still with us, of orthopaedic surgery and traumatology. So in spite of the criticisms that have been levelled at S.I.C.O.T. – and inevitably in the course of fifty years there have been a considerable number – despite the imperfections of all perfectible things such as S.I.C.O.T., I can say from a purley personal point of view that it has performed a most valuable function in giving me countless friends all over the world. So that I can say with the greatest conviction: I believe in S.I.C.O.T. And you?

Acknowledgements

I would like to extend may warmest thanks to all who helped me to prepare this booklet. Books, articles, photographs, personal archives, written and verbal recollections, documents, reprints, etc. ... have all been most generously entrusted, given or lent. There are far too many for me attempt to give a list of all those who co-operated in this task; I would be sure to leave someone out. So instead I would like to thank everyone, personally and individually, for their help. I am specially indebted to Miss LINDSAY WATSON, who has helped me in a wonderful way for the translation.

VdE.

---

* Paraphrase of Sir HARRY PLATT (The Eleventh Moynihan Lecture, University of Leeds, 25 May 1961, in "Selected Papers"; see note 11).

International
Orthopaedics

SICOT

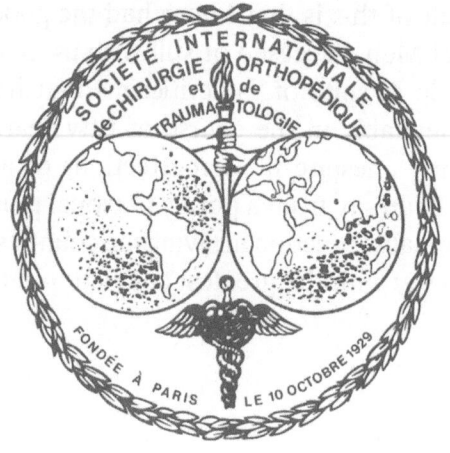

Official Journal of the Société Internationale de Chirurgie Orthopédique et de Traumatologie

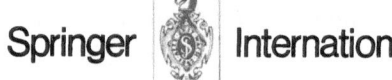

Springer International

144

International Orthopaedics
Official Journal of the Société Internationale de Chirurgie Orthopédique et de Traumatologie

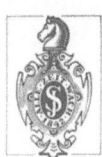

Springer-Verlag, Heidelberger Platz 3, D-1000 Berlin
Springer-Verlag, Neuenheimer Landstraße 28–30, D-6900 Heidelberg
Springer-Verlag New York Inc., 175 Fifth Avenue, New York, NY 10010

145